TRAIN *Happy*

AN INTUITIVE EXERCISE PLAN FOR EVERY BODY

Tally Rye

PAVILION

CONTENTS

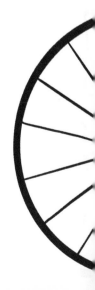

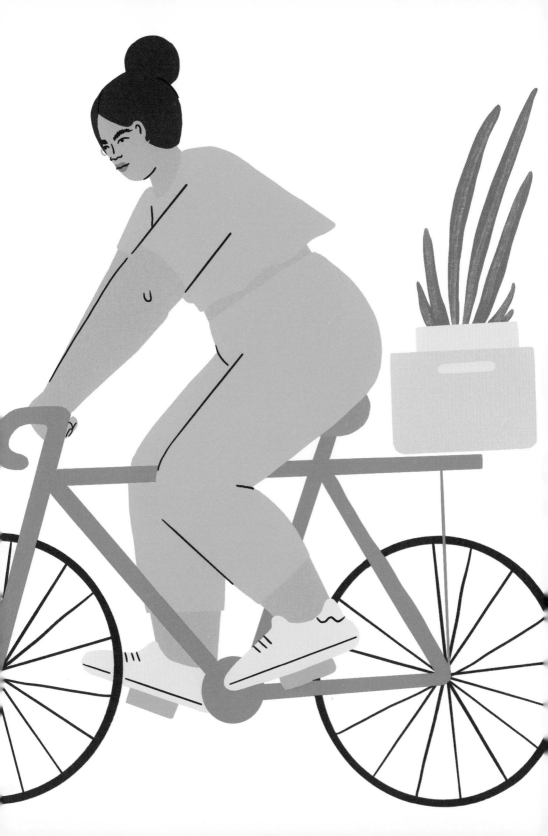

WHAT IS THIS BOOK ABOUT?

If exercise had ZERO impact on your weight and appearance, would you still work out? If you answered 'YES', would you work out any differently from how you do now? Would you do more or less?

In modern society, exercise has become synonymous with weight loss and aesthetics. In fact, I did a poll on social media to ask you guys whether you had initially started exercising for weight loss and aesthetics, or to feel good. Of the 2,314 people who responded, 81% said they initially started to work out as a way to manipulate their appearance. I wasn't surprised, because I too started my exercise journey thinking it was a sure-fire way of getting the body of my dreams. Growing up, I learned that exercise is a thing people do when they want to lose weight, maintain weight loss and counterbalance what they eat. My understanding was that it wasn't enjoyable, but it's just what you had to do to get the physique you really wanted.

This way of thinking about exercise and fitness urges us work out to achieve #bodygoals in a way that often seems arduous, painful and difficult, so many are put off because it doesn't seem like a fun way to fill time. And so, because fitness has become so intertwined with the pursuit of the leaner, lighter 'dream' body, the multitude of other benefits that an active lifestyle can bring have kind of been forgotten, or somehow seem less important. But they're not – they're hugely significant in the context of your physical and mental wellbeing, and so I've written this book to give them the airtime they deserve and to give you another perspective on what health and fitness are.

When aesthetic results are the primary motivation for working out, this is actually associated with less consistent engagement in physical activity, as well as worsened body image[1]. So, in this book, we are going to reassess what drives you to get moving. I want to help you build trust with yourself and reclaim your body so that you can enjoy exercise on your terms, in your own unique way. Because fitness can be fun, it can be something you look forward to and enjoy doing! Once you've finished reading this book, I hope you are chomping at the bit to explore all the wonderful ways there are to be active, and my workout guide (see page 86) will give you some clear guidance on how to get going.

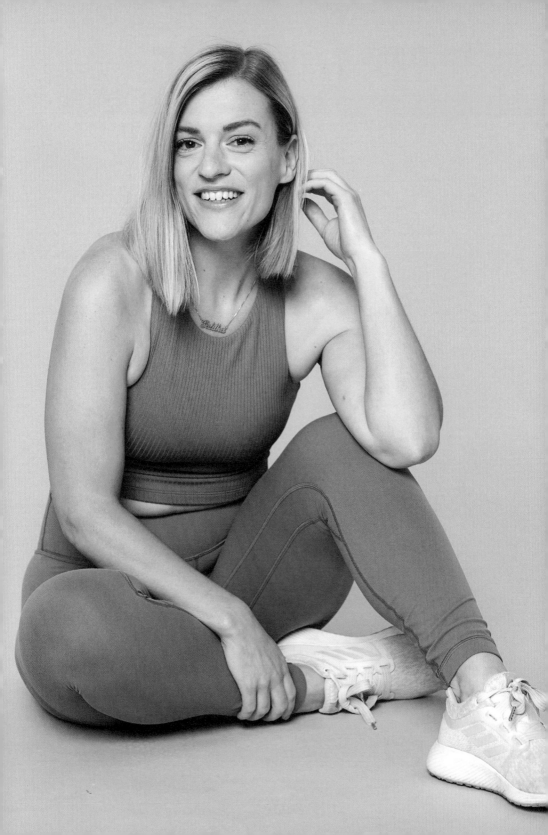

MY STORY

Up until the age of 18, I had little to no interest in fitness or nutrition, and I was pretty okay with my body. I didn't do sport, I struggled to run a mile and I ate whatever I liked. Then I started to pursue a career in musical theatre.

I spent the next five years at drama school in full-time training, trying to become the next big thing to grace the West End. With hardly any prior experience in performing, moving every day in front of a mirror in form-fitting outfits came as quite the shock. You can probably guess what the popular topics of conversation among the girls were: how to lose weight, good and bad foods, how to get visible abs and (shocker) boys! The thought process was, if we were slim we would be successful. The sad part about that assumption is that it was likely to be true.

Initially I felt like I'd been hit by a truck after the daily dance, stretch and body conditioning classes, but soon I got into the swing of things and actually started to enjoy the physical aspect of my potential career. See the thing was, I was a good singer and an okay actress, but a mediocre dancer. I tried my hardest in dance class, but I knew the one thing I could work on outside of class was my health and fitness. And so, I began to take on the identity of the 'fit' one.

Gradually, I became aware of my body in a new way. I thought I needed to be a size 8 and have a six-pack to even stand a chance of becoming the leading lady I'd dreamed of, so I paid closer attention to my diet than ever before.

In my second year, I began to develop gut health issues, which were eventually diagnosed as IBS. After very little guidance from my GP (but that's a whole other story), an online search led me to a wellness blogger's website, who was a leader of the 'clean-eating' crusade back then. She had similar symptoms to mine, and had cut out refined sugars and gluten and ate clean, so naturally I did too. Thus began the next phase of my food and fitness journey: the obsession.

At the same time, I vowed to exercise more outside of my daily dance classes. I graduated from home workout DVDs to a gym membership and discovered weight training for the first time. Crucially, this coincided with upgrading my phone, installing Instagram (my account was then called @cleanfitlifestyle), following #fitspo pages and scrolling through Pinterest for more #bodygoals motivation, workouts and recipes. I had unlocked a whole. New. World.
The fitness landscape on social media at the time was largely made up of bodybuilding and bikini competitions, progress pics and LOTS of perfectly presented food. I loved it. No one in my 'real life' cared about what porridge combination I had invented or what I had done at the gym... but the internet did! I felt like I'd found my tribe and, in some ways I had, because I've made some lifelong friendships through those social media connections. I discovered macro

counting and food tracking apps, I found out what a Bulgarian split squat was and prepped all my meals to eat from Tupperware. My goal was to get fit and healthy, and I understood that to mean dieting and getting lean. So, I spent my summer break working out six days a week, cooking 'clean' recipes and sharing it all online using hashtags like #beastmode #teamnodaysoff and following strangers around the world who were doing the same.

When I went back to college for my final year, I was ripped. I was so lean that when we had to do sit-ups in class it bruised my back. I was cold **all the time**. Not to mention totally preoccupied with tracking all my food. But did I mention I was lean?! And when I posted photos on Instagram of my perfect food and my six-pack, I felt validated as I got more likes and my follower count grew.

But I couldn't maintain this, it was all-consuming. And so, after a teacher expressed concern about my weight loss and behaviour, I started to think twice about what I was doing. Remember, it all started with me just trying to improve as a performer. I decided I would stop tracking my food and 'listen to my body' instead. But in reality, even though I was no longer using an app, I was still doing the mental maths. Letting go of rules around food and exercise was to be my battle for the next five years. The next phase I call: learning to relinquish control.

Six months after quitting tracking food I met my boyfriend. We started dating, and each time we met up it would challenge me to get out of my comfort zone a little more – whether it was eating ice cream out the tub for dessert, going out for drinks or doing something fun and missing a workout. It was uncomfortable at first but, ultimately, I enjoyed having more fun and being social.

After drama school, I decided I would become a personal trainer as being a part-time performer and a part-time PT seemed to complement each other. (Ironically, I actually never auditioned for anything, my heart wasn't in it like it was for fitness.) Moving back home with my family to get my qualification, I suddenly had a lot less control over my own food and exercise. As I became more sedentary, I started to see changes to my body and it was hard not to freak out. I felt like I was losing a part of my identity, and going into the fitness industry I worried that my body needed to be 'perfect' to succeed. But I was between a rock and a hard place because I didn't want to go back to tracking and intense training. I distinctly remember feeling like a failure when, during PT training, I realized that my own weight and body fat percentage had gone up.

I started working as a personal trainer in a commercial gym in London at the end of 2014. I've never worked harder than I did that year, and the message was reinforced that I needed to 'look the part'. Earlier that year, I had met two of my now closest friends; Zanna Van Dijk and Victoria Spence. We created an online movement called #GirlGains to help unite like-minded women like us. We needed promotional imagery for the website, so booked ourselves a photo shoot for September 2015 and, for the first time in a few years, I went back on a formal diet. I had a coach, and he gave me macros and a training plan to stick to.

But this time around, I had to maintain my job, relationship and a social life whilst prepping ALL my food and fitting in the workouts. Prioritising this regime above the people I loved meant I had to be selfish, and it put a huge strain on my relationship in particular. But even after 12 weeks of sacrifice, when the shoot rolled around, my body hadn't really changed. I couldn't help but compare myself to the other girls and feel inferior. Afterwards I just wanted to cry. At this point, my body image and confidence were at their lowest. Social media had created a fitness body ideal that I just felt I didn't live up to.

That was my last formal dieting experience. However, I've flip-flopped between living my life and wanting to be lean quite a few times since. There was that time when I did #projectreignitin because I wanted to get back some control around food. Another time, I had a nutritionist and personal trainer help me become my #BestMe, which really meant smaller me for an upcoming holiday. And when I shared this type of 'let's all get back on it' content online, my behaviours were praised. Even working within the fitness industry, I was confused by conflicting recommendations that asked me not to trust my own instincts. I was constantly fighting against my body to meet an aesthetic ideal that I now understand is simply unattainable for most people. When I learned that the majority of dieters fail (which we'll soon discuss in greater depth), I was shocked. No wonder I couldn't maintain such dramatic weight loss.

Over the past few years, I have made huge strides in healing my relationship with food and my body. Slowly but surely, I have been transitioning to a more intuitive mindset. Things really clicked when I discovered the book *Intuitive Eating*, by dietitians Evelyn Tribole and Elyse Resch. Their 10 principles have been an integral part of my journey to self-acceptance. Subsequently discovering intuitive movement has also opened up a whole new way of approaching fitness. Though this did not happen overnight, now I would say that fitness is an important part of my life, but not my whole life. I look forward to my workouts as a form of self-care for body and mind. I love food and it no longer has power over me – I don't know what I weigh, and I don't care.

By researching and digging deeper into myself, I have become free. I didn't realize just how oppressive my quest for the perfect body was. It stopped me from thinking, from being present and from connecting with people on a deeper level. For me, writing this book has been a testament to what I can achieve when I am at peace with my body and mind. I hope that it will help you get there too.

UNDERSTANDING DIET CULTURE

Understanding what diet culture is really helps give context to the ethos of *Train Happy*. You may well have heard the term banded about online and recently it has become a bit of a buzz word, but what does it actually mean? Well, it's the messaging centred around the belief that in order to be happy, successful, fit, healthy and attractive you must be slim. Being slim has also become equated with moral superiority. Praise is given to those who lose weight (regardless of the methods). And so, the reverse follows that if you're fat, you are shamed into thinking that you are unattractive, weak, lazy, unfit, unhealthy and a failure. Diet culture is rooted in, and perpetuates, fat phobia, which is a fear of fatness, of becoming fat and an intense dislike or hatred of fat people. It's a concept that has infiltrated our collective consciousness, we're taught these beliefs and views from a very young age – that ultimately fatness should be avoided.

Diet culture therefore encourages us to pursue a thin beauty and body ideal, because we never feel good enough and worthy enough of living our lives to their fullest if we are not meeting its (often naturally unattainable) standards. We are constantly fed messages that life will happen when we weigh X or fit a certain dress size, and many of us believe that. I certainly believed that. During those years at drama school, I held that to be absolutely true.

An obvious example of diet culture is all the various diets themselves. Diets take many forms, but really, they all want you to do the same thing: restrict to lose weight. Perhaps you have engaged in the following at some point: calorie counting, macro counting, points, syns, keto, intermittent fasting, cutting out carbs or dairy, clean eating, Special K, Atkins, detox plans... to name just a few. Don't worry if you have, it's extremely common! A study conducted in 2016 by a group of retail analysts found that in the UK alone, 48% of adults considered themselves to be on a diet. When analyzing the women who took part in the survey, 57% of those asked said they were on a quest to lose weight[2].

But this preoccupation of achieving the dream body is keeping us distracted and removed. As Naomi Wolf wrote in her book *The Beauty Myth*:

'A culture fixated on female thinness is not an obsession about female beauty, but an obsession about female obedience. Dieting is the most potent political sedative in women's history; a quietly mad population is a tractable one.'

This quote explains why it's so important that we recognize diet culture in all its forms, and call it out for what it is, in an act of defiance against patriarchal beauty standards – in other words, feminism.

So, why has our society become increasingly obsessed with achieving these beauty and body standards? Well, there is plenty of money to be made by creating 'flaws' and selling us the solution. In 2017, the global diet market was valued at just over $175 billion, with a projection that by 2022 it will be worth over $245 billion[3]. That's A LOT of profit being made from our insecurities. There are products such as skinny teas, waist trainers, juice cleanses, detox plans and meal replacement shakes being sold on the high street. There are the diet books, celebrity DVDs, TV shows, slimming groups, apps, online guides and meal prep companies, all there to help you with your 'transformation'.

Then there are the slightly more subtle but widely prevalent examples of diet culture, that sneakily infiltrate our thoughts and behaviours, perpetuating weight stigma. Maybe you've had or witnessed conversations that included things like: 'I ate take away last night, so I need to burn it off at the gym today' or 'I'm having a salad as I'm trying to be good'. This kind of stuff turns up everywhere, particularly in a fitness setting. 'New Year, new me' health kicks are another classic example of diet culture in action. They are often intense, unsustainable and short lived. This is how diet culture works – it's an industry that designs products and programmes that they know will eventually fail. It's a great marketing technique as it puts all the blame and onus onto us for not executing correctly; and so we buy into the next thing and the cycle continues. But I've written this book to tell you that it doesn't have to be that way AT ALL!

WHY DIET'S DON'T WORK

The big lie of diet culture is that it makes us think that losing weight and staying slim is simply the result of willpower and control. I asked Laura Thomas, nutritionist and author of *Just Eat It*, to explain why it's not that simple.

Popular narratives about weight suggest that if we burn more calories than we eat, we can successfully lose weight. This is known as the 'calories in vs. calories out' model. There are lots of permutations of this model, but they all 'work' by creating a calorie deficit. However, these simple equations belie the complex physiological and psychological processes that take place in our bodies when we restrict our calorie intake below our body's needs, meaning that, in the long-term, most people are likely to regain lost weight.

The idea that 'diets don't work' is not controversial among nutritional scientists;

we have long known that people can lose weight successfully in the short term, but that maintaining the loss is often difficult. Estimates on the failure rate of diets vary from study to study, which is why it can sometimes be helpful to pool a few different studies together into one larger study called a meta-analysis. One such study analyzed 29 randomized control trials of long-term weight loss and found that more than 50% of weight lost was regained after two years. After five years, that number was up to 80%. A more recent meta-analysis looked specifically at commercial weight-loss programmes (like Slimming World and Weight Watchers) and found that on these types of programmes, almost 60% of people failed to lose 5% of their body weight in the first place. These findings suggest that 1) it can be difficult for people to lose weight initially and 2) most weight loss is likely to be regained in the long-term. We are told that diets fail because of a lack of willpower, however weight regain is not a function of our resolve, it happens because of biological processes taking place in the body.

Let's first look at the physiological changes that occur when we diet or try to lose weight. Our body does all it can to defend what is known as our set point weight; our biological blueprint for the weight that is optimal for our bodies (in terms of our hormones, energy levels and immune function). Instead of being a specific weight, it is more accurately thought of as a range that our body will fluctuate between. For instance, it may go down if we are sick and can't eat, or up slightly if we have an injury and can't move around as much. When we try and push our weight down below this optimal range, our body will make adaptations to try and keep it within those limits. It is thought that as much as 75% of our weight is down to our genetics – contrast that with height which is 80% genetics – but we never hear of the 'get taller diet' - that would be ludicrous!

So, how does our body defend our set point weight when we go on a diet? Firstly, it does this by making changes to our appetite. People who are restricting their intake may have higher circulating levels of the hunger hormone ghrelin – this is an evolutionary mechanism to get us up off our butts when food is scarce. In practical terms this may mean that our cravings intensify, and we might feel preoccupied with thoughts of food and end up spending half the day googling recipes that fit our meal plans. On the flip side of this equation, we may also become less sensitive to our fullness cues – this is because of lower circulating levels of fullness hormones like leptin. This means we'll feel less satisfied after our meals and like we are never totally full.

On top of changes to our hunger and satiety cues, there are changes to our metabolic rate; it slows slightly to help conserve energy; our bodies can't tell that we're in a voluntary food deficit, it just assumes that food is scarce. For each kilogram of weight lost, our metabolism slows by about 20–30kcal/day, and our appetite increases by about 100kcal/day.

Not only do weight loss attempts tend to result in weight regain over time, but they may also be associated with higher risks of eating disorders and disordered eating. In a large study of 14-15-year-old adolescents who were followed up for three years, those who dieted 'moderately' had a five-fold increased risk of developing an eating disorder. The adolescents who severely restricted their energy intake and skipped meals were 18 times more likely to develop an eating disorder than those who did not diet. It's thought that dieting may also be related to binge eating, loss of muscle mass and strength, low mood (due to less serotonin production), anxiety, depressive symptoms and poor body image. What's more, dieting is, in and of itself, a predictor of future weight gain.

Although the evidence for this is less clear, it does seem that weight cycling (or yo-yo dieting) might be harmful for our health. Repeatedly losing and gaining weight might be related to more heart problems, worse blood sugar control, and poorer mental health compared to people whose weight doesn't fluctuate.

The relationship between weight and health is a lot less straightforward than thin=healthy, and fat=unhealthy. BMI is a crude measure of an individual's health, but it can be helpful in giving us some information about populations. Many people believe that there is a linear relationship between BMI and poor health; in other words, the higher the BMI, the worse health will be. However there is actually a 'J-shaped curve' between BMI and health outcomes. Let me explain – a recent study of over 3.6 million GP records from the UK found that those with a BMI of around 25 kg/m^2 (considered 'overweight') had the lowest risk of death and those who have a BMI ~ 30 kg/m^2 had a slightly lower risk compared to those who had a BMI ~18 kg/m^2. This tells us that weight, in and of itself, is not a great predictor of health; it doesn't provide the whole story.

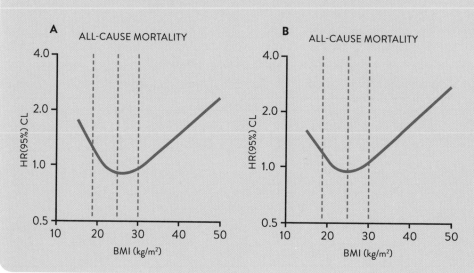

A more helpful measure of health risk might be to look at what's known as cardio-respiratory fitness – basically a measure of fitness level. Large meta-analysis studies have found that the risk of death from all causes (i.e. communicable and non-communicable) diseases is almost identical, regardless of BMI when fitness levels are high. Yup, people in the lowest BMI group ('normal') had the same level of risk as those in higher BMI groups. When fitness levels were low, however, the risk was double that of the fit group, but again, this was seen across all weight groups. The tl;dr here is that in this study, fitness was a more important predictor of health risk than fatness.

In another study of more than 12,000 Americans, researchers asked questions about four lifestyle variables thought to be important for overall health; not smoking, moderate alcohol intake, moderate exercise, and nutrition (five portions of fruit and veg a day). They found that when people didn't engage in any of the four behaviours, their risk of poor health outcomes was (unsurprisingly) highest, and the higher their BMI, the worse the outcome. However, when people in the highest BMI category engaged in just one of the health-promoting behaviours, their risk of death was cut in half. If people in the highest BMI category engaged in all four behaviours, then the risk was exactly the same as people in the lowest weight category. Again, this seems to indicate that health behaviours are more important for overall health than looking at someone's weight. And, although these studies are just observational, it also aligns with evidence from randomized control trials which suggest these behaviours are helpful, no matter your weight.

It's important to note though as much as 15% of our health status may be determined by our family history and genetic predisposition, which we have no control over. But by far the biggest contribution to our health outcome is our socio-economic status, accounting for around 50%. Health falls along a socio-economic gradient, meaning the poorest and most deprived in society are the most likely to have poor health-related outcomes; Public Health England estimates that people in the least deprived parts of England live, on average, 19 more years in good health than people in the most deprived areas. And even if people living in deprived areas engage in health-promoting behaviours, it's unlikely to be enough to make up for the disadvantage. The Food Foundation's Broken Plate report put this into context. If everyone were to follow Public Health England's Eatwell Guide, people in the lowest 10% of household income would end up spending 74% of their disposable income on food, and people in the most affluent 10% of the country would only spend 6%. While no one is disputing that nutrition can have an impact on health, we often forget to zoom out and put it into perspective with the wider determinants of health.

GET HAPPY

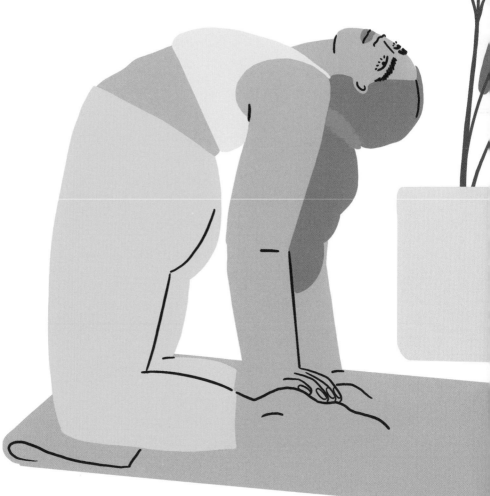

**How does exercise make you feel? Do you notice an
improvement in mood or confidence after you work out?**

When I ask people why they are initially motivated to start
regular exercise, the overwhelming answer I get is that they want
to change their body. But when I ask what keeps them driven
to regularly move their body, many say that the mental health
benefits are so significant that movement has become a key self-
care practice for them. And that is why this book is called *Train
Happy*. Above all, I want you to feel good – about movement,
about your body, about food and about your mind. The biggest
motivating factor in life is happiness – and I believe that, when
approached with a health gain mindset, exercise can be (one of)
many contributors to a more positive life.

In this section of the book, I hope we can learn more about
the importance of looking after our mental wellbeing, and how
exercise can play an important role in protecting and enhancing
the brain. Just as we aim to build a strong and fit body through
exercise, we need to put the same energy into building a
strong and fit brain. Our mental health is just as, if not more,
important than our physical health and so understanding how
we can support it is extremely important. As Dr Brock Chisholm
(the first director-general of the World Health Organization)
famously stated: **'without mental health, there can be no true
physical health'**.

We will also be exploring the links between body image,
happiness and mental wellbeing. Many of us look to body
transformations to make us happy and cure our bad body image,
but as we will discuss, the links are not so straightforward and
clear cut. By the end of this section, you will have more insight
into how to cultivate a healthy body image, acceptance and
happiness within your body, which will lead to more a positive
relationship with movement and exercise.

DIETS + MENTAL WELLBEING

We should never have to sacrifice our mental wellbeing in the pursuit of physical health, and yet sadly it is often collateral damage when pursuing intentional weight loss for aesthetic results.

As a teenager first embarking on my fitness journey, I was initially aiming for optimal physical health in order to become a better performer. At this point in time, I believed that 'physical health' had a certain look – slim, lean and defined. Due to my own ignorance, as I pursued this goal I didn't take my mental health into consideration. I focused intensely just on food and exercise, thinking that if I was slim and toned, 'healthy' looking, then that would automatically make me more successful and therefore happier. And whilst food and exercise may well have had a seemingly positive impact on my physical health to start with, I became increasingly obsessed with the methods I was using to get there. I would sacrifice time, energy and resources in order to meticulously plan my meals and fit in my extensive workouts, all the while neglecting all the other things that contribute to true health and happiness: social connection with friends and loved ones, spontaneity and freedom with food and exercise.

The more my gym goals evolved from health to changing my appearance, the more I would analyze every inch of how my body looked. Yeah, it was cool getting stronger, doing pull-ups and squatting my bodyweight, but eventually the only progress that really mattered to me was what I saw in the mirror. But the more intensely I focused on my appearance, the more my body image suffered. This was the true result of diet culture, and as with many diets, I did initially get the 'results' I hoped for, but these practices of intense exercise and food control were completely unsustainable.

Sadly, we know that there are lots of stories similar to mine, as studies have shown that many who embark on diets go down a path of controlling behaviours with food and exercise. 35% of occasional dieters progress to pathological dieting, which is defined as an unhealthy calorie or food restriction (for example, cutting out whole food groups such as carbohydrates). 20–25% of those pathological dieters are known to progress to partial or full syndrome eating disorders – that means 1 in 4 dieters are at high risk of developing an eating disorder[1]. So many of us are just trying to get healthy and happy through dieting as diet culture has told us to, yet it can severely negatively affect our mental health. However, I'm here to teach you that it doesn't have to be this way. If we reprogramme our relationship with food and fitness, we can unlock the many benefits that come from engaging in healthy behaviours that support both our bodies and our minds.

EXERCISE + MENTAL WELLBEING

As we become more aware of the importance of mental health, it's essential that we understand more about what we can do to protect it. To gain more of an insight into how we can be proactive, I asked psychiatrist Dr Sarah Vohra how exercise and other lifestyle interventions can play a role in supporting our happiness and brain function.

HOW WOULD YOU DESCRIBE GOOD MENTAL HEALTH?

I think there can often be an assumption that to have 'good mental health' you have to be free from any negative emotions or never have experienced mental illness, but it is not as clear cut as that. Throughout our lifetimes, we all experience a broad range of emotions, from negative to positive, and this largely depends on what is going on around us, the experiences we have been through in the past and the friendships and relationships we hold. Sometimes there may be no obvious reason for these emotions. I see good mental health as a state of balance and a feeling of contentment with the different aspects within your life, from how you feel about yourself personally and your capabilities, to how your brain is functioning (your focus, concentration and motivation), to maintaining positive interactions with friendships, relationships and within the workplace.

HOW IMPORTANT ARE LIFESTYLE INTERVENTIONS, SUCH AS EXERCISE, IN SUPPORTING GOOD MENTAL HEALTH?

Lifestyle interventions are hugely important, and their positive effects are often underestimated. Whilst there will always be a role for the conventional treatments such as talking therapies, and in some cases medication, lifestyle changes such as eating well, moving more and prioritizing sleep will optimize our mental wellbeing in the long term. They may even make us more resilient and better able to cope if and when life stresses do hit.

WHAT IMPROVEMENTS DO YOU SEE IN PATIENTS WHO INCREASE THEIR LEVELS OF ACTIVITY?

For a lot of individuals, exercise is a good way of managing and relieving stress. We are leading busier lives than ever before, fuelled by the fact that we are connected in a way we weren't going back 10 or 20 years; exercise offers a respite from that intense busyness and a break from the rat race. Different forms of exercise offer different forms of relief, whether taking out your frustrations on a boxing bag or being mindful and present during a yoga class. For the patients I see, regular exercise has helped their mood and improved their self-esteem. It has enhanced their focus and concentration during the day, so that they can perform better in their studies or at work, and it has also helped to improve their sleep.

HOW CAN WE MAKE SURE WE MAINTAIN A HEALTHY RELATIONSHIP WITH EXERCISE?

I think it is important to consider the reasons why you are exercising. For many, exercise is unfortunately still seen as a tool for punishment: to 'earn that meal' or to 'slim down ahead of that holiday'. Getting caught up in this rhetoric means that we are blinded from what we actually stand to gain from exercise – the copious mental and, of course, physical health benefits – and it also means that the period of exercise is less likely to be sustained – we throw in the towel as soon as we lose the weight or land at our holiday destination.

To maintain that healthy relationship, we need to shift the focus away from exercise just being a way to lose weight or attain a particular aesthetic, to thinking about what we stand to gain from it, (mental clarity, improved mood, better sleep). Here are some of my tips for doing so:

- » **Stop creating rules around how often you should be exercising – a little movement each day is better than none**
- » **Don't get consumed by tracking your activity or calories expended as a marker of your progress, and instead focus on how you feel. Compare your mindset pre-exercise (possibly stressed, tired) to how you immediately feel after activity (energized, elated)**
- » **Stop viewing exercise as being time-limited to justify a certain food craving or slim down to a certain size, and instead commit to it long term**

WHAT OTHER TOOLS DO YOU RECOMMEND FOR IMPROVING GENERAL MENTAL WELLBEING?

Getting a decent amount of sleep is absolutely crucial for good mental health and should be prioritized. Even just one poor night can affect how we think, feel and behave the following day.

Also, limiting screen time and prioritizing real-life friendships and relationships. Stop trying to juggle everything and start communicating to others, at home or in the workplace, when you are feeling stressed or overwhelmed, and feel confident in asking for support.

THE MENTAL HEALTH BENEFITS OF REGULAR EXERCISE

Exercise is not a replacement for therapy and medication but, as Dr Vohra suggests, when undertaken mindfully it can provide important support to our mental wellbeing. It's certainly a useful tool to have in our self-care kits and gives us a way of proactively building mental health resilience. Let me explain further some of the ways in which exercise can have a positive effect on mental health.

IMPROVED MOOD

How many times have you been in a bad mood, felt annoyed or frustrated about something, then completed a workout and afterwards almost forgotten what you were so riled up about to start with? This reminds me of one of my long-standing clients, Sally (not her real name). We train at lunchtimes, and she often comes in pretty het up after a busy morning of meetings. Our 45 minutes together are ring fenced as headspace away from the office environment, and instead Sally gets to focus on investing some time and energy back into herself. As you can imagine, she leaves feeling much better, often remarking 'that was just what I needed'. And interestingly enough, a recent study[2] found that raising your heart rate and working at a medium intensity for anywhere between 10–60 minutes has a positive effect on mood, including decreased feelings of depression, hostility and fatigue. This is because after you exercise, the brain can increase the happy neurotransmitters such as dopamine, serotonin, noradrenaline and endorphins, which are the ones that make you feel good… yay![3] This shows us that workouts don't need to be overly long or intense for you to feel those mood-enhancing benefits.

BUILDING MENTAL-HEALTH RESILIENCE

It's not just the short-term, immediate benefits to our mood that are apparent. Studies have shown that people who are highly active over long periods of time are less likely to develop depression due to the raised serotonin levels that exercise brings about[4]. Making an effort to move more, whether simply a walk outside on a sunny day, working out at home or attending a sweaty spin class, is a great way to get out of a negative headspace and distract from damaging self-talk. In addition to this, if you are able to get out to classes, running clubs or work out with a friend, this is a great way to feel a sense of community and belonging through real life interaction – a key component to positive wellbeing.

Often when people consider using exercise as a tool to support mental health, the first thing that comes to mind is an intense workout like boxing where you can punch the stress out. But fast and furious doesn't always equal most effective. As you build attunement between your body and mind (which we will learn more about later), you can learn to select the right type of movement for your personal needs so as not to add additional stress and pressure. For example, the gentler practice of yoga helps to regulate stress responses through techniques such as movement, meditation, relaxation and social connection[5] and so can be just as powerful in its own way.

IMPROVED SLEEP

Just one night of poor sleep can have an impact on our mood and energy the next day. I don't know about you, but my fuse is a lot shorter when I don't get adequate sleep, and I certainly feel less resilient to anything tough life might throw at me. However, increasing general activity levels and incorporating regular exercise into a weekly schedule have both been shown to have a positive effect on sleep and, more specifically, the quality of sleep. People who regularly exercise apparently sleep for longer periods without waking and have deeper non-REM sleep (the deepest part where you don't dream).

But what does this mean for mental wellbeing? Well, enjoying more good quality sleep means we have more energy to give a better performance when exercising, which releases more happy-mood hormones such as endorphins and serotonin. Quality sleep is restorative for the brain, which is important for maintaining good general mental health. Even more importantly, it builds resilience to diseases of the brain such as dementia, Alzheimer's and conditions like depression that sadly affect the lives of too many.

So, hands up who is aiming to get their 8 hours tonight and every night for the rest of the week? Sleep expert Dr Matthew Walker recommends going to bed at the same time every night and setting your alarm for the same time each morning to get a stable sleep pattern going. He also advises allowing yourself a window of time to get 8 hours of sleep every night, which means possibly 8.5–9 hours of rest time in bed to get the 8 quality hours of sleep required. Something I am always trying to work on!

IMPROVED COGNITION + BRAIN HEALTH

In her book *Healthy Brain, Happy Life,* Dr Wendy Suzuki proclaims that 'exercise is the most transformative thing you can do for your brain today!', which is a pretty bold, but exciting statement.

In her popular Ted Talk, 'The brain-changing benefits of exercise' (which I highly recommend you watch), Dr Suzuki shares her scientific findings. She tells us that a single workout can improve our ability to shift focus and attention and increase reaction speed times. Meaning we can be more productive when studying or at work, and the first one to run when the zombie apocalypse comes... okay, that last one I was just teasing 😉 but if you have exams or have a big work project coming up, be sure to stay active so that you can keep your brain razor sharp.

To reap the long-term benefits for the brain, Dr Suzuki recommends working out 3–4 times a week and raising your heart rate for roughly 30 minutes a session. This boosts the size of the hippocampus, a small but very important part of the brain that looks after your long-term memory, meaning you'll have clearer and more vivid memories, pretty cool right?! The research also suggests that keeping the hippocampi (there are actually two of them in your brain) and your prefrontal cortex (the bit of the brain behind your forehead) big and strong through exercise can help prevent and create resistance to degenerative diseases such as Alzheimer's and dementia, meaning it takes longer for these to have an effect[6, 7].

The brain health-boosting benefits of exercise are extremely significant and should not be underestimated. I hope this inspires you to move your body to support your brain for long-term optimal function.

MAKING TIME FOR YOU

If you've read this far, you'll know that exercise is an important component in protecting our brains and improving our emotional state (if you skipped straight to this part, just take my word for it). Exercise is just one piece of the larger health and happiness puzzle, so what else can we do to promote happiness and wellbeing?

You may have heard of the phrase 'you cannot pour from an empty cup'. So many of us try to run on empty because we give to others without giving back to ourselves, which inevitably leads to us to not showing up at our best or resenting even showing up at all. Putting energy back into yourself through self-care practices plays a massive part in improving both physical and mental wellbeing. And it's about so much more than just having a bath or putting on a face mask. It is about knowing when to stop, setting the boundaries in life that we are all entitled to and protecting ourselves from burnout.

Research professor Dr Brené Brown says that setting boundaries is 'about having the courage to love ourselves, even when we risk disappointing others', and that 'only when we believe deep down that we are enough, can we say "enough!"'. These are both powerful statements to reflect upon as they acknowledge that putting yourself first can involve uncomfortable situations where you have to say 'no'. But, Dr Brown argues, if we are brave enough to withstand these short moments of awkwardness, it will save us from spreading ourselves too thin and prolonged feelings of annoyance or bitterness.

For some, setting boundaries is easier said than done, as our economic situations often leave us with no choice but to juggle more than we can handle.

However, start small and do what you can. Even little, quick adjustments can make a significant difference to the energy with which you operate, helping you to slowly fill that cup back up. These acts also signify that you are worthy and deserving of time, which can in time strengthen your resolve until you become more assured with setting boundaries.

I encourage you to write down all the small ways that you manage to make time for yourself in the coming weeks and months, so you can look back and reflect on what felt good and get an accurate picture of how much time you allow yourself. Use the list below as a starting point and add things that are specific to you, your needs and your life.

SELF-CARE STARTERS	MY SELF-CARE LIST
» Adequate sleep (7–8 hours a night)	» _____
» Spending time with loved ones	» _____
» Time for hobbies	» _____
» Reading a book or watching a movie	» _____
» Regularly scheduled time for exercise/ movement	» _____
	» _____
» Rest and recovery	» _____
» Eating regularly	» _____
» Talking to a counsellor	» _____
» Going to therapy	» _____
» Laughter	» _____
» Meditation	» _____
» Saying NO to things – respecting your boundaries	» _____
	» _____

BODY IMAGE

I know on a personal and professional level that a desire to exercise is often connected to how we feel about our bodies. How we view our bodies can have an impact on our happiness and mental wellbeing, because it contributes to overall self-esteem. For some, body image is just part of what makes up their self-worth, but for many, living in a looks-obsessed culture, it's a significant proportion. People with positive body image and healthy self-esteem have a strong sense of self-worth, believing that they deserve love, care and respect. People who have poor self-esteem are often very critical of themselves, focusing on mistakes and weaknesses, believing they are inferior to others.

The aim of this section is to explain how exercise can make you feel *proud* of your body rather than coming from a place of feeling inadequate. I want to rid you of the toxic mindset that says looking slim is the only/best way to be body confident, and tell you that you don't need to rely on the scales, your dress size or your reflection in the mirror to feel comfortable in your skin.

EXERCISE + BODY IMAGE

Being motivated to work out from a desire to change your appearance is nothing to be ashamed of. Exercise has been sold to us this way for decades and diet culture and the fitness industry profit billions from your body hang-ups. The rhetoric can be roughly summarized as: 'when you change your physical appearance, you will feel good about your body, reach your potential in life, be loved, successful and live out your dreams…' And so, we start exercising with the aim of getting leaner and lighter, regardless of whether we are getting any enjoyment from the activity. Hands up if you've put yourself through a gruelling workout, despite hating the exercises (burpees, anyone?) but pushed through it anyway? Me, I have 🙋. Prior to these workouts, the old me would tell myself 'this one is meant to get me abs', and I would force myself through it. Afterwards, I'd step on the scale and check my abs in the mirror – and guess what? Nothing had really changed. Does this all sound familiar to you? Well, focusing on appearance goals didn't work for me, and I've since found research that shows just how detrimental it can be. Here are the headlines:

1. It actually makes us <u>less</u> likely to stick to regular training long-term[8].
2. It makes us feel rubbish about our body image, as we likely won't be able to change ourselves in the idealistic way we had hoped[9].
3. Those who engage in exercise purely for aesthetics are at a higher risk of developing disordered eating, symptoms of depression and lower self-esteem.

These findings are why I now advocate for the focus of exercise to be on how we feel within our bodies, rather than looks. When we make enjoyment and happiness the goal, it is likely that we will be able to be more consistent in what we do and develop an intuitive and trusting relationship with our bodies. Only then can we reap the awesome physical and mental health benefits of physical activity. I understand this won't be straightforward for everyone, but I hope that this book will help you get there eventually. Because, ultimately, our own mental health is more significant than making our bodies more palatable for society.

TASK

A positive way to improve your body image is to take pride in what it can *do*. Whether it's lifting weights, running a certain distance or becoming more flexible in yoga practice. Mentally or physically fill in the blank below:

I am proud of my body when _____
_____
_____

BODY POSITIVITY

You may already be familiar with the body positivity movement. It has gained huge popularity on social media, with people celebrating their bodies no matter their size. Consequently, it has been adopted as a buzzword by companies, gaining commercial success too. However, it was originally born out of the Fat Acceptance movement started in the 1960s by fat, queer, black and Jewish women. This was a political movement centred around social justice, it aimed to challenge society's systemic hatred of fatness and the anti-fat bias larger people encounter daily. The body image issues these women faced came from the external abuse and oppression they got simply for living in larger bodies.

As it has gained popularity over the past 10 years, body positivity has evolved. Today, it has become centred around fighting back against the narrow beauty standards of society and raising up those who have been widely under represented, particularly plus-size people of colour in mainstream media. On an individual level, it has had a huge impact with helping people learn how to love the skin they are in, despite the messages they receive from wider society.

Personally, I love this message. I believe we ALL deserve to experience body acceptance and respect, though for some of us that is easier than others. I support the Fat Acceptance and body positive community, but I do not try to centre myself within it, instead I aim to be an ally. Why? Well, I'm a slim, white woman and that comes with a lot of privilege. I have certainly had body hang-ups and body image issues, but I don't face the same struggles that those living in bigger, marginalized bodies do on a societal level. When I watch TV and read magazines, there are plenty of people who look like me. I can find clothes that fit me in any high-street store, and I can go to the doctors without being told to lose weight despite having an unrelated health concern. No one judges me for what I eat, or tells me I'm a drain on society simply from looking at my body. My body type is already widely represented and accepted – body positivity is fighting for those who are not. In its truest form, it is wonderful – lifting up those who really need it and giving people who feel left out a place to belong.

BODY ACCEPTANCE

With the rise in popularity of body positivity and its links to self-love has come the pressure to love yourself, love your body and love your appearance no matter what. But if you have felt uncomfortable in your body for a long time, or have been fighting against it, using food and exercise as weapons, the idea of loving or even liking it might feel a million miles away from where you are right now, and that is more than okay. Shifting a mindset from hate to love is a pretty huge and rather daunting challenge. If that feels too overwhelming, I'm about to introduce you to some ideas that can help. Body acceptance is a key tool that you can use to make a positive shift towards using exercise as a form of self-care and health gain, rather than punishment. To find out more, I spoke to body acceptance coach Kristina Bruce to discuss how it can help us.

HOW DO YOU DEFINE 'BODY ACCEPTANCE'?
Firstly, I should begin by saying that body acceptance shouldn't be viewed as resignation or 'giving up' on caring for our bodies. On the contrary, our ability to truly care for our bodies becomes possible when we are in a place of acceptance rather than struggling to change. From this place of acceptance, we can tune in to what our bodies (and mind and spirit) need in order to feel nourished and fulfilled, rather than basing this on trying to meet an external standard.

I define body acceptance as focusing on caring for our bodies and living our lives without trying to drastically change them to fit a cultural ideal. For most of us, this looks like moving and eating in a way that brings nourishment, pleasure and ease. It looks like being okay with (or at least neutral about) our bodies. It's understanding that our bodies will change – that they are not meant to stay or look the same. And it means doing our best within life's circumstances, knowing that we are valuable and worthy no matter the look or ability of our bodies.

HOW DO YOU EVEN START TO ACCEPT YOUR BODY?
We all have various experiences of living in our bodies. Some of us are struggling with a chronic illness or disability. Some of us have been shamed for not looking a certain way or being unable to perform to a certain level of expectation.

The intensity of these experiences can be painful and challenging to live with. However, if we refuse to accept our bodies or our circumstances, we stay stuck thinking about 'what ifs' or yearning for how we looked in the past.

I always ask the question: 'what does not accepting your body cost you?'. For many people, not accepting their bodies costs them peace of mind and the ability to be able to enjoy what they can in the moment. It keeps people closed off to possibilities. It costs us the joy of wearing the clothes we want, being present with our kids, enjoying a delicious meal or the money and time spent on weight loss programmes. When we see that not accepting our bodies costs us so much, it can be the catalyst that we need to start learning to accept our bodies.

Another important thing to note is that what we have come to view as an 'beautiful' body is actually nothing more than cultural conditioning. We all grew up with a constant barrage of messages from family, friends and television of what an 'ideal' body looks like. We are told that certain bodies are 'better' than others. But this ideal is not fact, it's a belief – and beliefs can change. We know this to be true when we look across cultures and history to see that beauty ideals everywhere are different and always changing. But truly, any ideal ends up excluding someone, so the move towards accepting that bodies come in all different shapes and sizes, with their own inherent beauty, will better serve us all.

HOW CAN BODY ACCEPTANCE IMPACT OTHER AREAS IN LIFE?

When we can accept our bodies, we release a lot of stress and anxiety that we may not even realize we are carrying. We are able to let up on the subtle (or maybe intense) criticism that we play over and over in our minds when we feel our bodies should be different. Overall, we'll feel more energized and healthier, because instead of forcing our bodies to do exercise that is punishing or not eating enough food, we are fully nourishing our bodies with food that we enjoy and allowing for more rest and ease. We open up more time in our day that might have been taken up by exercising or counting calories to spend with friends and families or have fun engaging in activities we enjoy.

Furthermore, when we are so critical against ourselves, we tend to act this way with others, so we may find that our relationships improve when we more fully accept ourselves. We may find that we're more easily able to let things go that aren't in our control and move with the flow of life. And as we become more accepting, we open our hearts more, so we'll often become even kinder and more loving towards ourselves and others. Life in general becomes a bit easier.

BODY NEUTRALITY

I first came across the idea of body neutrality a few years ago when I was training a client who listens to a podcast I host, called 'Fit & Fearless'. The particular podcast discussion had been about body image and body positivity, to which my client remarked 'But why do I have to love my body? Why can't I just feel neutral about it? Or indifferent? Why does it have to be such a big deal?'

She was right, why indeed? Discovering how to feel neutral towards my body has helped a few missing pieces fall into place for me. I struggled to love and accept my body 24/7 and was almost fed up of thinking about it all the time. When I realized that body neutrality only asked me to feel indifferent about my appearance, and further, not really focus on how I look at all, it really resonated with me. Before this revelation, I had existed in an echo chamber of body positivity and self-love. I assumed that we all wanted to and *had* to love our bodies because that was the only option. I now realize that I don't need to love my body all the time to be able to treat myself with care and respect.

I believe that a big part of the journey to body acceptance is understanding that the body you inhabit is merely a home for the other gifts that you possess – things like personality, kindness and intelligence. That particular realization was a moment of release for me. All the time and energy I used worrying about how I looked could be put into nourishing me as a person; reading more, laughing more, gaining greater life experience instead. In my early twenties, I was so focused on shaping my appearance that I could never have written this book. I didn't have the headspace, the energy or the self-belief. So, understanding that my worth does not lie in my weight has given me the freedom to go beyond skin deep and dig deeper into *who* I am as a person. I now want to nurture the gifts I have in order to make a positive impact on this world. I asked Anuschka Rees, author of *Beyond Beautiful* and advocate of body neutrality to tell us more.

HOW DO YOU DEFINE BODY NEUTRALITY?
Body neutrality is about reducing the enormous significance that's being given to physical attractiveness in our society.

WHAT'S THE DIFFERENCE BETWEEN BODY NEUTRALITY AND BODY POSITIVITY/SELF-LOVE?
Body neutrality goes beyond body positivity on both a systemic level and individual level. Systemically, body positivity has focused on challenging society's narrow idea of beauty – which is necessary. However, we also need to push back on the aspects of society that make adhering to those ideals seem significant in the first place. On an individual level, whereas body positivity typically focuses on helping people feel good about the way they look, body neutrality is about helping them internalize that they are so much more than the way they look.

WHAT CAN WE DO TO FEEL MORE NEUTRAL TOWARDS OUR BODIES?

It's about recalibrating your self-worth barometer and understanding that the way you feel about your looks is not the marker for how to feel about yourself or your life. It requires actively training yourself to focus on positive, non-appearance qualities. For most people, this constitutes a huge mental shift, requiring education and reflection to question your own self-talk and why you feel the way you do. And it's not just that our thoughts influence our actions, our actions influence our thoughts as well. Some helpful actions are:

1. Don't engage in negative self-body talk among friends and family
2. Unfollow any social media accounts/influencers that make you compare yourself to them or bring you down when you see them
3. Fill your social media news feeds with accounts that inspire you for reasons other than health and beauty inspiration
4. Do activities and exercises that are fun and make you FEEL good, rather than those that help you achieve a certain look
5. Remove any steps in your beauty routine that feel like a chore. Keep the ones that feel like a good use of your time

HOW CAN WE NAVIGATE A WORLD THAT IS BODY-OBSESSED?

One important thing we can do is change how we talk about beauty and looks. In our culture, it's so ingrained in us to compliment women on their appearance, even female newborn babies get told they are pretty, whereas baby boys get told they're strong, even when they look identical. The same thing happens with adult women, so a first important step is to pay attention to how you talk about women you meet or see on TV and try to divert your speech away from their outfits or their body. Instead, talk about what they are saying or doing or their personality instead. The second step is then to apply that same non-appearance-based language to yourself. For example, when you see a picture of yourself from a party, don't talk about the way you look, talk about how fun that party was. Use your language and your attention to help internalize the idea that you don't equal the way you look.

IS IT OKAY TO NOT EVER LOVE YOUR BODY?

Yes! And in my opinion, this notion that one needs to love their appearance at all times in order to be happy is just another reflection of the overvaluing of beauty in our society. Just look at young children – socialization tends to hit them while they are still confident and running around on the beach without a care in the world. Their happiness doesn't come from them thinking their thighs/stomach/face are looking great – it won't even have crossed their minds! Yes, you should strive to cultivate respect for yourself as a human being, and your body is a part of that. But, if your main goal is to be happy and feel confident, understanding that you are more than your body is the most valuable thing.

ACCEPTING AN EVOLVING BODY

As we begin to accept our bodies and become less controlling with food and exercise, our appearance may change, and that can feel disconcerting. Wearing a bigger dress size can trigger a desire to diet and get back to your former body. When I first started to relax my approach to diet and exercise, my body slowly changed. I had been at a low weight my body wasn't happy with, and it was fighting back to restore me to the optimal size it knew I would thrive at. But I didn't trust it, because diet culture had told me that fit, healthy and acceptable looked like the cover of fitness magazines. But in reality, my body isn't meant to fit that mould, and very few people naturally are. Here are some valuable lessons I have learned that have helped me come to accept these changes.

Bodies come in all shapes and sizes – We are not all meant to look the same and we are not all meant to wear the same dress size. We never question that some people are tall and some are short, that some have big feet and some have small feet. We also accept that some people are naturally thin. So why do we struggle to accept that some people are naturally fat? Bodies are diverse and we all have the right to take up space in this world. **Stop comparing to your past self** – Our bodies will evolve and change as we go through life, we will not look 21 forever and nor should we. We are constantly moving forward, dealing with the cards that life hands us, and our bodies will reflect that. You don't have to look like you did at prom, or like you did on your wedding day or before you had children. Changing is not failing – our evolving and fluctuating shape is part of the human experience, so embrace it and remember all the incredible things that your body has done for you. **Stop comparing to others** – Someone else's existence, does not lessen yours. Anuschka Rees spoke about avoiding this in the context of social media, but when you find yourself comparing your body to others in real life, firstly remember all the wonderful things about you that don't relate to your appearance. Secondly, shift the focus and put your energy into enjoying the task at hand. Perhaps you're on the beach, so go for a swim or read a book. Maybe you're on a night out – go for a dance and sing along to the music. **Wear clothes that fit** – Wearing old jeans that dig in and feel super tight will quite literally make you feel uncomfortable. But wearing clothes that fit your new shape will help you to feel at ease in your skin and move freely, allowing you to just be present in your body.

We are all being held back because we are struggling to accept our bodies. But accepting your body, feeling neutral or even loving it, is a radical act! It's putting up the middle finger to diet culture and the companies and businesses that profit from making you feel insecure and not good enough. Diet culture wants to keep you small, subdued and pre-occupied. When you push back against that and live a big, loud and purposeful life – YOU are the one that profits!

SOCIAL MEDIA

Within the discussion of body image and mental wellbeing, I am fascinated as to how social media has had an impact – it exposes us to a lot of stuff that we weren't really privy to just 10 years ago. I'm a millennial, so social media is a big part of my daily life and I'm assuming it may well play a part in yours too.

Social media often gets a bad rep with regards to mental health, and understandably so, as overexposure to it seems to cultivate negative feelings. The trouble is, it can make it seem like everyone else has it all – the job, the holidays, the well-behaved kids, the 'perfect' figure. How many times have you had a scroll through and felt worse about yourself afterwards? It's not surprising that being exposed to hundreds, maybe thousands of people's highlight reels every day makes us feel like crap. It's a comparison trap, particularly when it comes to body image.

The rise of #fitspo on social media has made the fitness community even more image obsessed. It has become a place to show off #bodygoals, before and after photos and make body comparisons. Regardless of the captions, we are drawn to the imagery first and foremost. We scroll through and click on hashtags, often only seeing a narrow body type as fit, attractive and accepted and wondering how everyone eats the most perfectly presented meals 24/7.

I myself used to spend hours on these platforms, finding recipes, workouts and following women whose bodies I admired. In the end, it did lead me to look like them for a little while, but as I explain early on (see page 7), I couldn't sustain those behaviours, and trying to do so was damaging to my mental health. The more I consumed content, and compared my body to my peers, the more I felt like I came up short. I find it quite ironic that despite being at my leanest, and having people online tell me I looked great, I felt more uncomfortable in my body than I ever had before. That was my experience, but I am fascinated as to what the research says about the effects of social media on our body image, so I spoke to body image researcher Nadia Craddock to find out more.

ARE THERE LINKS BETWEEN SOCIAL MEDIA IMPROVING OR WORSENING BODY IMAGE?

Personally, I don't think social media is inherently bad for body image, but there is a lot of content out there that can be harmful to it, such as heavily filtered and edited idealized images of people's bodies. There is also some content in particular that is extremely concerning, such as pro-anorexia type content and influencers pushing the skinny/detox teas that are prevalent online. There are many studies now that point towards the idea that the more time we spend on social media, the worse we feel about our bodies[10]. But when we unpack this a little, this link seems to be contingent on *how* we use social media.

Specifically, the following appearance-focused activities on social media are associated with negative body image[11]: **following accounts that only show very idealized, unrealistic pictures of people's bodies**, particularly if we find ourselves comparing our (unedited and unfiltered) bodies to these images and (almost inevitably) finding ourselves falling short. **Spending lots of time and effort selecting and editing pictures of yourself** – for them to be 'good enough' – this process can increase body image anxiety and body shame via self-objectification – the act of viewing ourselves from an external perceptive focused on appearance, rather than other values and emotions. Finally, **viewing or making appearance comments on other people's photos** – when we read or write comments like '#bodygoals' or 'you've lost so much weight, you look amazing', our attention focuses on appearance. This can pull us back into the appearance comparison trap and leave us feeling more self-critical.

Given that social media is not going anywhere, researchers have been exploring whether anything on social media can help people feel better in their bodies. Although this research is still very much in its early stages, there are some encouraging findings. For example, one study found that viewing 'body positive' content on Instagram (where posts promote body acceptance, celebrate bodies that do not align with society's traditional narrow appearance ideals, and critique narrow appearance ideals) was associated with improvements in young women's body image and mood[12]. Being critical of the media we consume is a powerful, well-established mechanism for disrupting the pathway between viewing idealized images and negative body image as it reminds us that aspiring to change our appearance is a distraction and a burden on our resources (time, money, energy) and as such is disempowering, particularly to women.

Another study found that viewing side-by-side images with a thin-ideal model image and a parody image (Celeste Barber) imitating the model was associated with improvements in body image and mood in a sample of young women compared to viewing thin-ideal model images alone[13]. Through humour, these images may help us rationally process these images as unrealistic. A third study found viewing self-compassion quotes on Instagram (e.g., 'you are doing better than you think', 'be kind to yourself') was associated with improvements in body image and mood among young women. This study found that viewing self-compassion quotes in amongst fitspiration images seemed to buffer the negative impact of the fitspiration images[14]. Also, a couple of studies have found viewing pictures of nature have prompted small short-term improvements in body image[15].

HOW DOES #FITSPO HAVE AN EFFECT ON FEMALE BODY IMAGE?

This is interesting because although #fitspo appears to be promoting health, the images in #fitspo content are typically still thin and toned, and there's a strong focus on the appearance-related benefits of exercise and fitness[16]. Perhaps unsurprisingly then, research has found that viewing #fitspo content on social media has a negative effect on women's body image, mood and self-esteem[17]. These effects were felt amongst women who had a greater tendency to compare their appearance with the #fitspo images.

One study[18] that I think is really interesting in the context of fitspo is when researchers looked to see if viewing #fitspo led to an increase in exercise in real life. Not only did the study find that viewing #fitspo images (from google and Instagram) increased women's body image concerns, it found that although women who viewed these images said that they were inspired to exercise more, this did not translate to actual increased exercise in real life. **That is, viewing fitspo posts of the stereotypical thin and toned women did not promote greater physical activity, it just left women feeling slightly worse about their bodies.** This study also found that women who viewed the fitspo ideal images reported higher body dissatisfaction scores compared to those who viewed the thin ideal images. It's suggested this might be because with fitspo, there is the implicit message that you could look like this if only you worked hard enough.

HOW DOES BODY IMAGE AFFECT RELATIONSHIPS WITH EXERCISE?

In general, people who exercise seem to have a slightly better body image than those who don't[19] and exercise frequency is positively correlated with positive body image[20]. It's likely that this relationship works both ways. For example, participating in exercise seems to reduce body dissatisfaction[21] and, particularly when there is a focus on the health and enjoyment benefits of exercise, it seems to also contribute to positive body image[22, 23]. It is also possible, however, that people with a positive body image are more likely to exercise for health and enjoyment in the first place. It's often the case that people with poor body image have a complicated relationship with exercise and are more likely to either over or-under-exercise[24].

HOW DOES SOCIAL MEDIA ENCOURAGE SELF-OBJECTIFICATION?

It's difficult not to be drawn into self-objectification when we are viewing endless photos of other people and curating our own. Self-objectification is the process in which we view and critique our appearance from an external perspective. According to Objectification Theory, this constant self-scrutiny and monitoring of our appearance can lead to body image concerns as well as depression and disordered eating[25]. Some of the mechanisms of social media (e.g. likes) can intensify own self-scrutiny of the images of ourselves, as we are reminded that our images are being evaluated by external viewers[26].

CAN YOU GIVE US SOME EVIDENCE-BASED IDEAS ON HOW WE CAN IMPROVE OUR OWN BODY IMAGE?

Yes, I've listed some below. It's also good to remember, though, that body image is a personal experience, so it's worth exploring what works for you.

1. Being critical of oppressive, unrealistic beauty ideals and toxic messages about appearance that are pervasive in society
2. Learning about the social justice component to body image: although body image is an internal psychological process, it is informed by the patriarchy, white supremacy and fat phobia
3. Practicing activities that foster a greater connection between mind and body – yoga is a good example, as is dancing or life drawing
4. Self-affirmations and reminding yourself of your value beyond your appearance
5. Practice mindfulness and self-compassion. Don't beat yourself up for not 'loving your body' enough. Let it go and be kind to yourself
6. Stop engaging in body talk about your own body (e.g. I hate my arms) or other people's (she's so skinny). Even positive-sounding statements like 'you've lost weight, you look great' can have a negative impact. Set boundaries with your friends and family and talk about something else

In the context of social media, the best thing to do is curate your feed:

1. Unfollow accounts that makes you feel bad about your body
2. Follow accounts that promote body acceptance and celebrate bodies that do not align with society's traditional narrow appearance ideals[27]
3. Follow educational, social justice accounts that critique society's traditional narrow appearance ideals as oppressive
4. Follow non-appearance-based accounts that are aligned to your actual interests beyond your body. They will remind you that you are more than just your body
5. Parody images (such as Celeste Barber) mocking unrealistic, objectifying images may be helpful[28]
6. As can accounts that post self-compassion quotes[29]

Nadia Craddock has given us such great insights from the research. Now we need to put it into practice in real life. I have shared a list of resources at the back of this book (page 156) to help you foster better body image and body neutrality. We all have a much greater purpose, and I hope this section helps you take a step closer to realizing what yours is.

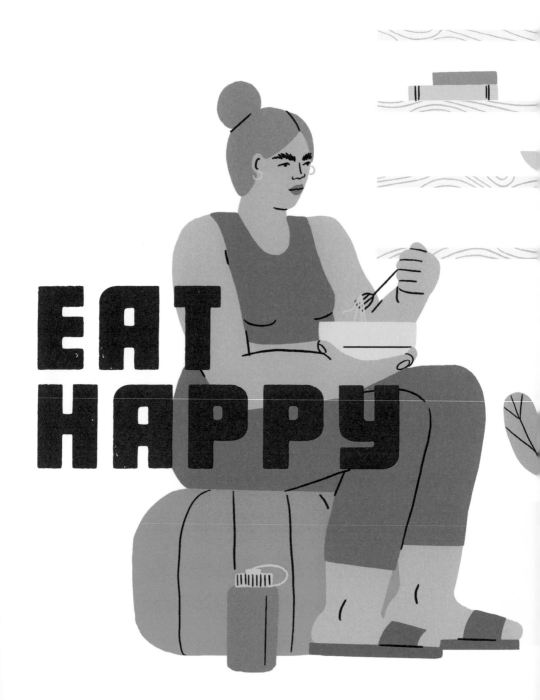

What is a fitness book without some mention of food or nutrition? It seems that these two things come hand in hand, which is understandable given that both behaviours are pieces of a big puzzle that makes up our overall health.

However, in modern society the lines between training and food have become blurred, meaning that personal trainers, like myself, are often thought of as nutrition gurus too. I'm honestly not quite sure how that happened!? But I do have my theories. Exercise has become so synonymous with weight loss that much of the fitness industry has felt pressure to deliver dramatic body transformations in order to be seen as successful. And a key component of weight loss? Diet and calorie deficit. Training alone often cannot achieve such dramatic results. Therefore, the industry has adapted to try and offer the complete package to people, whether they are fully qualified to or not. It's becoming increasingly normalized that fitness trainers will provide detailed nutrition advice through meal plans and macro calculations. But for the majority of those working within the industry it is out of our realm of qualification to do so. A two-day course learning about Nutrition for Fat Loss is not the same as a Nutrition or Dietetics Degree – trust me, I did the two-day course!

While all this might seem like just a response to client demand, it has been recognized as a great way to make money and adopted as a key marketing strategy. The diet industry is reportedly worth $176 billion dollars worldwide[1] and the fitness industry is cashing in by offering services which are often outside of their scope of practice. The fear is that by not giving the training AND nutrition information to a client, they will not be satisfied and take their business elsewhere. As a consequence, even though this is primarily a fitness book, I felt that it *had* to cover the topic of food and nutrition, because it has become so widely expected by you, the reader, and the wider industry.

So as a consumer and potential client, please be wary of who you get your nutrition information from and don't be afraid to ask questions about qualifications. You deserve to receive help and guidance from the best qualified practitioner. I recommend working with a degree-level educated nutritionist or dietitian for the best care possible. My hope is that it becomes commonplace for fitness professionals to work alongside nutrition professionals, who do have the relevant qualifications, so they can provide the best, and safest, service possible as a team. So that's what's about to happen right here!

But if I'm not going to write about food for fat loss – what is this section going to be about?! In the pursuit of health and wanting to have the perfect diet to yield perfect 'results', things have become a bit messy and complicated along the way. We have become so focused on *what* to eat that we don't reflect on *how we feel* about what we are eating. Diet culture has had a strong external influence over what we deem to be the 'right' or 'wrong' things to be consuming. Therefore, I want to use this section (with the help of a dietitian) to instead get you thinking about **your relationship with food** and how it makes you feel.

RELATIONSHIPS WITH FOOD

My relationship with food was a significant part of my overall fitness journey, and perhaps it is for you too? All the various rules I imposed on myself lead to a big level of distrust between my mind, body and food. I endeavoured to have the 'perfect' diet that would give me the 'perfect' body, but it led me to exhibit controlling and disordered behaviours that are becoming all too common. Some of these showed up as:

> » Logging everything I ate into an app and feeling anxious if I didn't
> » Only feeling comfortable eating the foods I classified as 'good' and 'clean'
> » Having to know the calorie and macronutrient content of any foods before I ate them
> » Struggling to eat outside of my routine or be spontaneous – looking up restaurant menus in advance to make sure there was something I could eat before going
> » Working out to counterbalance the guilt If I ate food I deemed as 'unhealthy'
> » Using a fitness tracker to tell me how many calories I could eat in a day (no more than I had burned)
> » Never having a dressing on a salad for fear of extra calories, and always having sauces on the side
> » Never 'drinking my calories' and always ordering water
> » Having to present my food to look perfect and 'Instagrammable' for every meal or snack

As you can imagine, this put strain not only my relationship with food, but those around me too. It was hard to eat out, to be cooked for and to attend events if I didn't feel in control of the menu. Diet culture had told me that if you enjoy food, you have to burn it off. I used exercise to justify or negate eating and it was a balancing act. Therefore if there was an imbalance, it could send me to a negative place of guilt and shame.

What's more, the more I learned about food (mainly from questionable sources online), the more I became confused and overwhelmed as to what the 'right' way to eat was. Was it low-carb? Was it high fat? Was it macros? Should I be intermittent fasting? Or going keto? This was my story, but we all have our own relationship with food derived from our own experiences. Our narratives are influenced by a wide range of factors from relationships and life experiences. I would like you to take this opportunity to reflect upon your own journey so far; what are the beliefs you already have about food? And where they come from?

WHAT IS A NORMAL RELATIONSHIP WITH FOOD?

We've discussed how diet culture has caused our relationships with food to become skewed over the years, so now I want to expand on what a positive and normal relationship with food may look like. We praise people for eating 'healthy', thinking that is what we should all be aiming for. But, so often, we understand 'eating healthy' to mean restricting food in some way. So, what does a normal relationship with food look like? In her 1983 book, *Secrets of feeding a healthy family*, dietitian and psychotherapist Ellyn Satter described it in the following way, which I believe still rings true today:

» Normal eating is eating competence. It is going to the table hungry and eating until you are satisfied

» It is being able to choose food you enjoy and eat it and truly get enough of it – not just stop eating because you think you should

» Normal eating is being able to give some thought to your food selection so you get nutritious food, but not being so wary and restrictive that you miss out on enjoyable food

» Normal eating is giving yourself permission to eat sometimes because you are happy, sad or bored, or just because it feels good

» Normal eating is mostly three meals a day, or four or five, or it can be choosing to munch along the way

» It is leaving some cookies on the plate because you know you can have some again tomorrow, or it is eating more now because they taste so wonderful

» Normal eating is overeating at times, feeling stuffed and uncomfortable. And it can be undereating at times and wishing you had more

» Normal eating is trusting your body to make up for your mistakes in eating. Normal eating takes up some of your time and attention, but keeps its place as only one important area of your life

» In short, normal eating is flexible. It varies in response to your hunger, your schedule, your proximity to food and your feelings

INTUITIVE EATING

It may be helpful to take a moment to think about where you are at in relation to the description on the previous page of a 'normal relationship' with food. If you feel that you are not at this place, then please be kind and compassionate to yourself, what I'm about to tell you about will help.

So much of diet culture is about gas lighting. It makes you believe that you cannot trust your own instincts and you don't know the best way to care for your own body. Intuitive eating is a revolutionary concept which fights back against this. It's not another diet with strict rules about what to eat and when. You don't have to cut anything out, measure, track or fear food. No. It's all about you rebuilding trust with your body so that you can get back to your natural instincts – the ones you had as a child when you knew what food you liked, how much of it to eat and to stop when you'd had enough. Discovering intuitive eating was a game changer for me. It has challenged so many of the rules and beliefs I had about food. Now I can be spontaneous again and enjoy delicious meals and snacks without guilt. It has given me unconditional permission to eat food regardless of exercise. And it taught me how to honour my health and wellbeing without having a strained relationship with food. The concept has 10 key principles which help to guide a process of building back trust with your body, ultimately giving the power back to you to decide what's best for it:

THE 10 KEY PRINCIPLES OF INTUITIVE EATING

1. Reject the diet mentality
2. Honour your hunger
3. Make peace with food
4. Challenge the food police
5. Feel your fullness
6. Discover the satisfaction factor
7. Cope with your emotions
8. Respect your body
9. Exercise and joyful movement
10. Gentle nutrition

As Evelyn Tribole, co-author of the book *Intuitive Eating* says, **'intuitive eating is a personal process of honouring health by listening and responding to the direct messages of the body in order to meet physical and psychological needs'[2].** Each person's path will be different, but ultimately it empowers you to take back charge of your own body. I asked registered dietitian (and certified personal trainer) Jessi Haggerty to more formally introduce us to the concept of intuitive eating and break down the key principles:

The concept of intuitive eating was developed in the 1990s by two dietitians, Evelyn Tribole and Elyse Resch, and was designed as an antidote to the rise of fad diets during that time (a.k.a., the rise of the low fat vs. low carb debate). Tribole and Resch wrote the book titled *Intuitive Eating* (now in its third edition) and outlined ten principles to help their readers get off the diet roller coaster and have a more peaceful relationship with food.

The book's subtitle is 'a revolutionary program that works' however, intuitive eating is not really a programme at all. In fact, the mainstream refers to it as an 'anti-diet' and refers to the book's 10 principles as guiding lights rather than rigid rules to be followed. Clinicians like myself have used these principles as a foundation and often further customize the practice to meet the needs of the specific population or individuals they serve.

While there is no one 'right' way to be an intuitive eater, Tribole and Resch have made one thing very clear: Intuitive eating was and is not designed to be a weight loss programme. There have been over 90 studies performed to measure the positive outcomes of adopting an intuitive eating practice, and it has been hypothesized that one potential outcome is that your body will find its set-point range (the weight range your body wants to maintain for optimal function), but the bottom line is, this practice really has nothing to do with weight. The goal is to help you have a more peaceful, nuanced relationship with food.

I don't think we can talk about intuitive eating without first talking about diet culture. The first principle of intuitive eating is **reject the diet mentality**. Here's the thing about the diet mentality: you don't have to be on a diet to be trapped in the diet mentality, and that's because we live in a diet culture. We live in a culture that tells us we need to ignore and suppress our hunger (a.k.a. our biological need for food and survival), and pursue thinness and body perfection at all costs. Our inner 'food police' follow us around to criticize us for breaking the rules and making sure that every indulgence is followed up by a punishment in the form of guilt, shame or suggested compensatory behaviour like over-exercising or skipping meals.

This leaves us on this never-ending roller coaster of following the rules, breaking the rules, feeling guilty, paying penance, and starting fresh. And every time we go around another loop, we blame ourselves for not being able to 'stick with it' and lose sight of the fact that we can actually choose to get off the ride. But the problem is not that we lack willpower or self-control, the problem is that following the laws of diet culture often means ignoring the laws of physiology. Your body is not interested in diet culture. Your body wants to survive and thrive, and it can't do that if you don't *feed it*.

A simple (but not easy) place to start is with the third principle of intuitive eating: **honour your hunger**. This can be really difficult when diet culture has taught us to question our hunger by suggesting that perhaps we are just bored or thirsty, and that if you are feeling hungry the chances that you are, in fact, actually hungry are quite slim. Rejecting this notion and trusting your hunger might be challenging, but every time you trust your hunger signals and respond by feeding your body adequate amounts of satisfying food, you let your body know you are on the same team. It's important to remember that hunger isn't an 'on' or an 'off' state. You are not 'hungry' or 'not hungry', but instead likely experiencing a range of hunger at any given time. Practice noticing when your thoughts shift towards food, when your stomach feels empty, when the thought, sight or smell of food seems appealing, when you're feeling irritated or having trouble focusing. All of these sensations are signs of hunger and it's important to honour that, even if you feel like it's 'too soon' to eat again.

(**Author's sidenote:** When I first saw the hunger and fullness scale below as a visual, something clicked for me. For so long I had let myself get to almost totally empty before thinking I was allowed to eat again. Because of my intense hunger, I would then eat until I was uncomfortably full. Learning to spot my signs of hunger earlier on and honouring those signals means that instead of

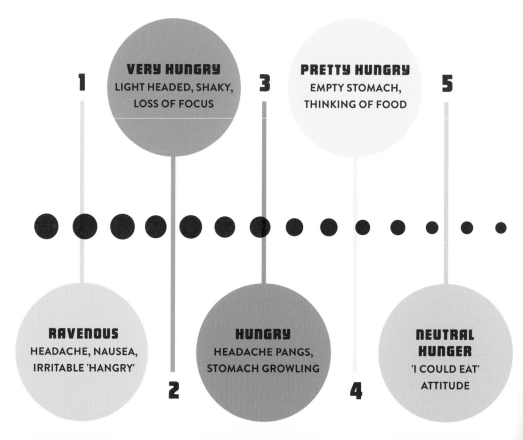

1

VERY HUNGRY
LIGHT HEADED, SHAKY, LOSS OF FOCUS

3

PRETTY HUNGRY
EMPTY STOMACH, THINKING OF FOOD

5

RAVENOUS
HEADACHE, NAUSEA, IRRITABLE 'HANGRY'

2

HUNGRY
HEADACHE PANGS, STOMACH GROWLING

4

NEUTRAL HUNGER
'I COULD EAT' ATTITUDE

the pendulum swinging from far left (1–2) to far right (9–10), finding the sweet spot in the middle (3–8) has kept my energy levels more balanced, and left me a lot less hangry!)

It's hard to talk about hunger without talking about fullness. The tricky thing about the fifth principle of intuitive eating: **feel your fullness**, is that worrying about 'getting too full' is a slippery slope back into the diet mentality, and if you're not careful, it can pretty quickly make you shift gears into a restrictive mindset. My favourite way to help clients with this principle is to teach it in conjunction with the sixth principle of intuitive eating: **discover the satisfaction factor.** We can work these principles simultaneously to honour our bodies physiological need for adequate calories, protein, carbohydrates, fat and fibre, while also honouring our desire to receive pleasure and satisfaction from food. The best way I can describe it is that feeling after you finish a meal when your stomach is full and you don't want any more of the meal in front of you, but you're on the hunt for something. Maybe it's something sweet, or something crunchy. Some might call this a 'craving'. This is not a malfunction on your part. Seeking pleasure from food does not mean that you are 'addicted' or 'out of control'. Food is supposed to be pleasurable, so enjoy it!

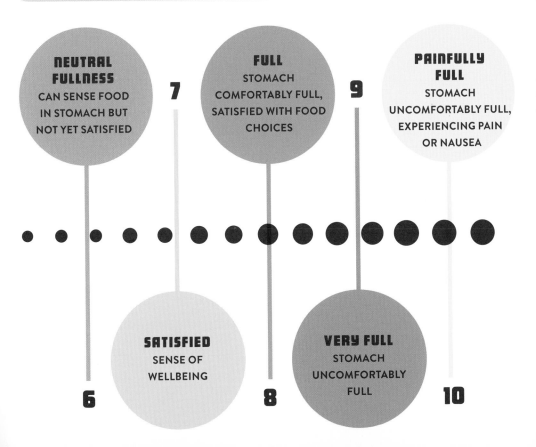

NEUTRAL FULLNESS
CAN SENSE FOOD IN STOMACH BUT NOT YET SATISFIED

7

FULL
STOMACH COMFORTABLY FULL, SATISFIED WITH FOOD CHOICES

9

PAINFULLY FULL
STOMACH UNCOMFORTABLY FULL, EXPERIENCING PAIN OR NAUSEA

SATISFIED
SENSE OF WELLBEING

VERY FULL
STOMACH UNCOMFORTABLY FULL

6

8

10

I know that enjoying food might be easier said than done. This is where the third principle of intuitive eating comes in handy: **make peace with food**. Throughout this process, it's going to be really tempting to try to put the brakes on your intuition. You'll be craving some chocolate and the whole time you're eating it the diet mentality will be whispering: are you sure you want to keep eating this? It's pretty sneaky like that. But making peace with food is about giving yourself **unconditional permission to eat.** This means that you can eat what you want without conditions. So, when that diet mentality pops up, just gently remind it that it's not needed right now because you have permission to eat what you want, when you want, and how much you want.

Like I mentioned above, intuitive eating is not a weight-loss programme. It's not a weight-anything programme. It truly has nothing to do with your weight. The eighth principle of intuitive eating is **respect your body**. This means embracing the body you were born with, in all of its iterations. Our bodies change from the day we are born to the day we die and it's a waste of precious time and energy to fight that. You can respect your body by practicing intuitive eating and you can also find your own unique ways to respect your body. Dress in clothes that feel comfortable and represent your unique style, move in ways that feel good for your unique ability level, make time to rest, and use your body as a vehicle to experience your life.

Now to answer the question everyone asks when it comes to this concept: But what about health? What about nutrition? Does that just go out the window? When you first start an intuitive eating practice, it might be necessary for you to put your definition of 'health' or 'nutrition' on the back burner while you do some of the deeper exploratory work. This might take a few weeks, months or years. It's truly different for everyone. The key to tackling the tenth principle of intuitive eating, **gentle nutrition**, is to eat in a way that supports your needs and not turn this principle (or any principle) into another set of rigid rules.

WAYS TO PRACTICE GENTLE NUTRITION

Switch from a mindset of restriction to a mindset of adequacy – Diet culture tells us that we need to live our lives on as little food as possible. But the reality is food is energy and we need to make sure that we are fuelling our bodies with the energy they need to survive and thrive. No more skipping meals, eliminating food groups from our diets, or over-exercising to compensate for eating.

Eat every 3–4 hours – Your body's quick energy stores deplete every 3–5 hours, so eating at regular intervals ensures that you'll have enough energy to go about your day and prevent extreme hunger. Try to have a balance of carbohydrates, protein and fat at these intervals if possible.

Eat a variety of foods – Once you get far enough along in the intuitive eating process, you'll realize that you no longer have to intentionally 'moderate' your intake. Your body will do the checks and balances for you. You can ensure nutrient balance by giving yourself access to a wide variety of foods, this includes fruits and vegetables but also includes fun foods like chips, cookies, and ice cream.

With this information it's important to stress that developing an intuitive eating practice is a slow-going process, especially if you have a history of dieting or disordered eating. If you're finding this information overwhelming, visit www. intuitiveeating.org and find a certified intuitive eating counsellor to work with to help guide you through this process.

WORKING TOWARDS A POSITIVE OUTCOME

Intuitive eating is a unique approach to nutrition because it focuses on us fostering a positive relationship with food. I believe it's so important to build this strong foundation of trust with ourselves as we navigate our own food journey and the research on this agrees: intuitive eaters are said to enjoy a more varied diet[3], as Jessi Haggerty recommends. It is also evident that intuitive eaters have greater body appreciation and satisfaction, better life satisfaction, psychological hardiness, positive emotional function and much more motivation to exercise when the focus is on enjoyment rather than guilt or appearance![4]. Later in the book we will be exploring the connected concept of intuitive and joyful movement in more depth and thinking about how we can apply the principles of intuitive eating to how we think and feel about exercise.

When we discuss food, it is important to emphasize that it is a privilege to make choices over what we eat and how we move our bodies, due to socio-economic status. Sadly, not everyone can afford the luxury of accessibility and choice, which is wrong and unfair. In the UK, the use of food banks is considerably on the rise. The charity Trussell Trust reports that from 2014–2019 food bank use has increased by 73%[5], and from 2018–2019 they delivered almost 1.6 million three-day emergency food parcels to people and families in need. For all of us to have the opportunity to build a more positive relationship with food, we need to think on a broader scale and fight for a more equitable society.

TRAIN HAPPY

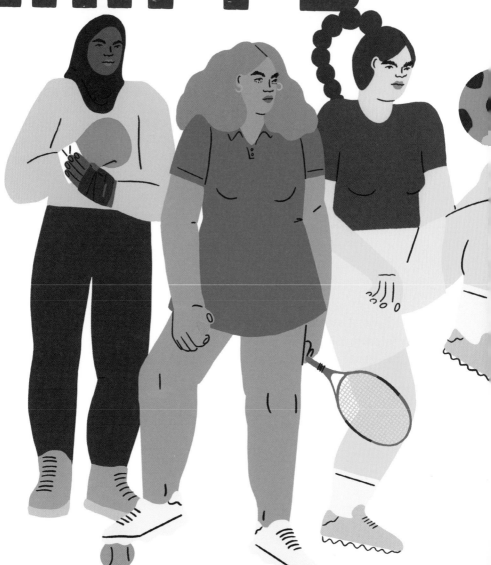

Now we get to what I call the really fun part! In this section we will be discussing the *Train Happy* mindset and approach to fitness. As diet culture only focuses on the weight loss and body composition aspects of fitness, in this section we well delve deeper into ALL the benefits of exercise, and reclaim movement as a way to feel good and thrive. We'll think about what constitutes a workout, and go through the different ways we can move our forms, inspiring us to think outside the box and have fun with fitness. I also want to teach you all about the concept of 'intuitive movement', which is born out of the intuitive eating framework (see page 38). We'll discuss how you can take practical steps to build trust with your body and cultivate a positive relationship with exercise. By the end of this section, I want you to feel more confident within a fitness setting and have the tools and knowledge you need to navigate your own path so that you can make the best choices for you.

SHIFTING MINDSETS

Both personally and professionally, I have transitioned from working and training with what is called a 'weight centric' approach to a 'weight inclusive' approach.

The **weight centric** approach is very typical of the fitness industry, with much of the goal setting focused around achieving the desired aesthetic through weight loss and muscle gain. These types of primary goals inevitably influence the narrative and language used in training, and it becomes strongly associated with those who want to visibly change their bodies. Examples of this include your standard '12-week body transformation challenge' or class instructors encouraging participants to 'burn off the weekend', perpetuating the idea that exercise is nothing more than another way to shed calories. Success through the weight centric lens looks like inches, pounds and percentages of body fat lost.

Through the **weight inclusive** lens, however, we don't look at what is lost through exercise, but instead what a person can holistically gain from taking care of their body and mind. This inclusive approach to training doesn't use weight, body measurements or aesthetics as a marker of progress, but instead focuses on improvement in various levels of fitness and enhanced happiness and mental wellbeing. The aim is to help you improve your quality of life through health-promoting behaviours, regardless of whether there has been a change on the scales. You don't just have to take my word for it, there is important research that shows that when we focus on exercise just as a form of self-care, it improves people's overall health and happiness regardless of weight or size[1].

The weight inclusive approach is aligned with and born out of the Health At Every Size® movement. As written on the ASDAH (Association For Size Diversity And Health) The Health At Every Size® principles are:

1. Weight inclusivity Accept and respect the inherent diversity of body shapes and sizes and reject the idealizing or pathologizing of specific weights.

2. Health enhancement Support health policies that improve and equalize access to information and services, and personal practices that improve human wellbeing, including attention to individual physical, economic, social, spiritual, emotional and other needs.

3. Respectful care Acknowledge our biases, and work to end weight discrimination, weight stigma and weight bias. Provide information and services from an understanding that socio-economic status, race, gender, sexual orientation, age, and other identities impact weight stigma, and support environments that address these inequities.

4. Eating for wellbeing Promote flexible, individualized eating based on hunger, satiety, nutritional needs and pleasure, rather than any externally regulated eating plan focused on weight control.

5. Life-enhancing movement Support physical activities that allow people of all sizes, abilities, and interests to engage in enjoyable movement, to the degree that they choose.

Though I sound clear cut in my approach now, my own shift in mindset did not happen overnight. When I first got into fitness, I too was sucked in by diet culture. I believed that if I wasn't losing weight, getting leaner and visibly seeing results then I wasn't doing it 'right'. Perhaps you have felt the same way? Therefore, I put myself through workouts I didn't enjoy, trained more than I really wanted and sacrificed other parts of my life to accommodate the gym. It was an exhausting lifestyle I couldn't maintain. If and when I fell behind with my intense workout schedule, it made me feel anxious about the changes that might happen to my body. However, I was excited at the idea of loosening the reins and having more flexibility and freedom to try new forms of movement. I didn't want to put so much emphasis on the aesthetic anymore, but that was all I knew fitness and exercise to be, and so changing my outlook took time. I'll share more about how you can work through that process later on.

Shifting the focus of my training to mental wellbeing, enjoyment and more performance-based goals, has taken the pressure off. It has given me a greater connection to my body, and I have been able to honour what it needs instead of insisting on training in a certain way as dictated by diet culture rules. It's been really fun to play at the gym again, to get outdoors, to enjoy new experiences in classes and learn new techniques. I'm having fun again, and I aim to bring that new energy into every other aspect of my life.

MOTIVATION

It's well known that staying active is generally good for you. But if we know this, why do most people still find it difficult to make time for regular fitness?

Two words immediately spring to my mind here: diet culture. As mentioned already, diet culture has turned exercise turned into something we do purely to lose weight and change the way we look, which is why many of us now associate it with unpleasant notions like discipline, restriction, punishment and pain. It's thought of as something we should endure in order to look a certain way. For many, despite endless burpees or miles on the treadmill, it still doesn't achieve the desired aesthetic we were promised. So, if it isn't necessarily going to make you look the way you really want to and it's causing lots of physical discomfort, then it's not hard to see why a lot of people struggle with motivation.

It's also worth mentioning here that some people who are naturally slim may have even less motivation to work out, because they already exist in a body that conforms to society's standards. We all have that friend who seems to 'eat whatever they want', not really work out and show no sign of weight gain. The messaging around working out, getting good sleep and eating more vegetables every day is that we do these things to keep ourselves slim; so if you're naturally small already, it might seem like a waste of time or something that isn't really for you. The privilege of existing in a smaller body means that less external pressure is felt to conform to society's standards. On the flip side, people in larger bodies are regularly shamed into exercise and told that they 'should' move more as a way to improve health. But in reality, ALL bodies, big or small, can benefit from an active lifestyle and everyone should equally be encouraged to do so.

EXTRINSIC MOTIVATION

This is when your motivation for moving your body and/or engaging in health behaviours comes from extrinsic (outside or external) influences. For example, you may be spurred on to work out and change what you eat because of other people's comments, because you feel pressure to conform to a certain body type or because it's what your favourite celebrity is promoting. Diet culture thrives off extrinsic motivation by creating 'flaws' and selling apparent solutions. The problem with using an external influence to motivate is that eventually it fizzles out. If you're engaging in a behaviour primarily to please others and not yourself, then it isn't going to last long term.

INTRINSIC MOTIVATION

So let's talk intrinsic motivation. This is when your motivation for moving your body comes from you. There is no deadline, you work out because you want to and not because you feel outside pressure to conform to the ideas and opinions of others. You do it how you want and when you want – basically, YOU DO YOU 🏃. The best way to develop intrinsic motivation is by educating yourself about the physical and mental health benefits of regular movement (see page 50) and learning which types of workouts suit your body and mind best. The aim is that you can find incentive to exercise as a form of self-care, self-respect and because it just makes you feel good. Cultivating greater intuition with your body is an important part of this process – if you turn down the volume on all the outside noise (extrinsic motivation/diet culture), your body will tell you that it needs different things at different times in your life.

Our reasons for motivation, chosen forms of movement, routine, amount of time and goals will change and evolve as we journey our way through life. I like to remind myself of this, as different things will take priority at different points in our lives. I have been fitter in the past, and I may well be fitter in the future, but right now I can commit to a level of exercise and activity that fits with this moment of my life. There is a tendency to panic if our fitness levels are not always on an upward trajectory, but as with life, they will ebb and flow. Remember to think of the big picture, and as the saying goes, life's a marathon and not a sprint.

We are in this for life, right? There is no deadline on being active. How you choose to move your body as life changes may look differently from year to year. That is okay. The best routine for you is the one you can consistently do at this time in your life. It never needs to be perfect, it just needs to be right for you.

MOTIVATIONAL LANGUAGE

As a lot of the fitness industry operates within the weight centric sphere, the motivational language you might be used to is often based around shame and guilt. You've likely seen quotes like this online or heard a class instructor say something similar to:

'Excuses don't burn calories'
'If you work hard now, you'll get that summer body'
'Work hard to earn that dinner'
'Press-ups get rid of your bingo wings'
'Burn off the weekend'

A study conducted by Northwestern University[2] brought to light how this type of language can affect us. Two groups of participants each took part in a 16-minute conditioning class. They did the same workout, in the same room, to the same music, but the instructor used a different script for each. For one group, the instructor used motivational language such as 'this exercise builds strength in the legs; these are the muscles that truly help you run, jump, sprint like a super hero!'. After the class, the female participants reported that they felt more positive about their bodies, and said they felt 'accomplished' and 'strong'. For the other group of participants, the instructor made appearance-focused motivational comments like, 'this exercise blasts fat in the legs, no more thunder thighs for us! Get rid of that cellulite!'. This second group of participants didn't share the same feeling of positivity after their workout. Instead, when asked to describe how they felt at the end of class, they said things like 'ashamed' and 'disgusted with myself'.

These results are the perfect way to illustrate how much better we feel after exercise if we're simply enjoying it rather than worrying about burning calories or striving for a six-pack. The moment you put all that stuff to the side, working out can make you feel so powerful and positive.

Have you ever heard of the phrase **'move because you love yourself, not because you hate yourself'?** I want to add to that phrase **'move because you RESPECT and want to CARE for yourself, not because you hate yourself or your body and want to punish it'.** When thinking about your own motivations to work out and move, ask yourself: where is this motivation coming from? How does it feel to move from a place of care versus moving from a place of punishment? Perhaps you may choose to do things differently.

THE BENEFITS OF EXERCISE

In the list below I've broken down many of the key benefits of exercise. From the pleasant perks of staying active to the astoundingly serious reasons for doing so, you may be surprised at the variety of the things you see. Note that not one of these 29 benefits is related to aesthetics or weight loss, which is routinely touted as the main goal of exercise thanks to diet culture. Distracting people from the more serious and important benefits of exercise does both your health and the fitness industry a great disservice, and I believe that better education and awareness in this area is vital. As we have already looked closely at the mental health benefits of exercise in the first section, let's dig a little deeper into some of the physical benefits.

PHYSICAL	MENTAL
» Increased sensitivity to hunger and fullness	» 30% less risk of depression (NHS)
» Improved posture	» 30% less risk of dementia (NHS)
» Reduced back pain	» Improved sleep
» Improved strength	» Improved self-esteem
» Improved cardiovascular fitness	» Sense of accomplishment and achievement
» Improved bone density	» Improved body image
» Helps prevent injuries	» Greater body appreciation
» Increased mobility	» Improved memory performance
» Increased flexibility	» Greater focus and productivity
» Increased stamina	» Better mood
» Lowers mortality risk (death rate)	» Helps manage anxiety
» 35% less risk of heart disease and strokes (NHS)	» Relieves stress
» 20% less risk of developing breast cancer (NHS)	» Provides social interactions
» 50% less risk of developing colon cancer (NHS)	
» 83% less risk of osteoarthritis (NHS)	
» 68% less risk of a hip fracture (NHS)	

MORTALITY

The big one. As morbid as it may seem to consider our own mortality, I think that most of us would be really grateful to live a long, full and happy life – and exercise is something that can help with that. We know that physically active people are generally much healthier than sedentary ones, regardless of their weight: A study conducted as part of the Aerobics Center Longitudinal Study in Texas[3] found 'obese' men, classified as 'fit' based on a treadmill test, had death rates equally as low as fit 'lean' men. Additionally, the men who were obese but fit had half the death rates of the lean but unfit men. They found similar results for the women. So, I encourage you not to wait to be a certain size before exercising... you can reap the benefits right now! Fitness is not just good for those who fit the lean *Women's Health/Men's Health Magazine* stereotype... it is and *should* be for *every body*!

FUNCTIONAL STRENGTH + QUALITY OF LIFE

And on the theme of improving your quality of life, it's so empowering when you feel strong enough to carry all the groceries or to pick up a heavy box, or when you feel energized enough to clean the whole house and play in the garden with the children in your life – this is functional strength and fitness in action! I asked my community on Instagram to share some of the ways that functional strength gained through fitness has improved their quality of life, here is what they said:

'More patience, resilience and perspective to deal with what life offers'

'Ability to open jam jars'   'Feeling calmer in myself'

'Able to help people with their bags and suitcases on public transport'

'More energy for long and regular dog walks'   'Much easier to walk up stairs'

'Better posture when sitting at my desk at work'

'More focused when exercising before work'

'Greater lung capacity to sing all parts of Bohemian Rhapsody' – my personal favourite!!

This is a great opportunity to note down the ways in which fitness has positively impacted your life. Write down three or more (non-appearance-related) benefits that you've felt and take a moment to reflect upon their significance to you. Come back to this section if you're ever having moments of doubt or feeling confused on your fitness journey as you transition to a health-focused approach.

EXERCISE HAS HELPED ME _____

_____

_____

POSTURE + BACK PAIN

In recent years, we have become a much more sedentary society, with many of us travelling to work in the car, sitting at a desk all day, then going home to sit again. This lack of activity means depletion of muscle, which bears consequence on our posture. Bad posture looks like rounded shoulders or sticking your lower back and glutes out and poking the chin upwards. I'm pretty certain we all can identify with a few of these bad habits! Incorporating exercise, in particular resistance training, can have a positive impact in helping to strengthen our musculoskeletal system. The NHS recommends focusing on strengthening the core, back muscles and glutes to help reduce the risk of developing lower back pain in the first place, and as part of a rehabilitation programme that can help to reduce existing back pain and discomfort. Evidence suggests that working on core stability, training the glutes and dynamic stretching helps to reduce pain and disability for those with chronic lower back pain[4, 5, 6].

BONE DENSITY

Exercise, particularly weight-bearing and resistance exercise, is widely recommended as one of the primary preventative strategies to reduce the risk of osteoporosis; a condition that weakens bones[7]. It is most effective in people under 35, as from the age of 35 onwards our bone mass begins to decline. The American College of Sports Medicine recommends adults should aim to work out 3–5 times a week for 30–60 minutes to improve bone mineral density. They encourage a variety of weight-bearing endurance exercise such as tennis, jogging and stair climbing, jumping activities and regular weight training.

DIFFERENT WAYS TO BE ACTIVE

There are SO many ways to move your body! I use the phrase 'move your body' a lot in this book because it reminds us to keep our minds open to different activities outside of a traditional gym or fitness setting. Exercise is not just about pumping weights, doing HIIT or running for miles – it can be varied, fun and challenging in so many different ways. It's also important to acknowledge that a gym setting is not for everyone for multiple reasons – not everyone feels comfortable or welcome there. Others may not have the means to pay membership fees or afford access to the latest classes.

So, we need to be creative, open minded and accepting about the ways we choose to move. Let's let go of fitness stereotypes and think broadly when it comes to ways of getting active. Fitness can be fun, it doesn't have to be all sweat and muscle soreness. I know some think that a workout is only valid if it's in a gym setting, burns a certain amount of calories or raises the heart rate a certain amount – I spy diet culture coming by to ruin the party again!

WAYS TO MOVE YOUR BODY

RUGBY

BODYWEIGHT WORKOUTS

ROCK CLIMBING

DANCING

MARTIAL ARTS

WALKING

POWER LIFTING

ICE SKATING

NETBALL

HIKING

HORSE RIDING

PILATES

GOLF

ZUMBA

POLE DANCING/
POLE FITNESS

ICE SKATING

TRAMPOLINING

WEIGHT TRAINING

ROWING

YOGA

CYCLING

SKIING

RUNNING

FOOTBALL

This is your reminder that all of the activities above count. Some will be more strenuous, and others will be gentler, but they are all valid because they all involve moving your body. I would love you to think about trying a new activity from the list this month, or use it as inspiration to think about what other things you enjoy doing, and maybe get some friends or family involved!

Another type of movement we tend to overlook is the every day activities that keep us moving and mobile. If you are used to being pretty sedentary, then start with the list below and enjoy steadily increasing your daily activity before trying more formal types of exercise. That way, movement becomes habitual and part of your normal routine and your fitness levels will start to gradually improve. It's also good to remember the many simple ways we can get moving in our daily lives when we don't have time for an 'official' workout.

> » Take the stairs instead of a lift or escalator
> » Skip a step when walking upstairs... it's like a lunge!
> » Park further away from where you need to be and walk
> » Go for a longer walk on your lunch break
> » Take an evening sunset stroll
> » Walk or cycle to work if you can
> » Tend to your garden
> » Complete an energetic bout of housework
> » Get a coffee to go and enjoy a walk and catchup with friends

WHAT MAKES A GOOD WORKOUT?

It's simple, really. A good workout is one that you enjoy and can do relatively consistently over time. It's not necessarily the one that burns most calories, lasts the longest or gives you the most achy muscles. Of course, you can still do workouts that tick all these boxes, but they're pretty intense on the body and so it's not advisable to train to your maximum at every single session. You also don't need the added stress of attempting to fit in consistently rigorous workouts on top of busy modern life, as that will only increase the psychological pressure and be counterproductive in the long run. Instead of going full throttle every time, I encourage you to listen to your body and manage exercise alongside other factors such as sleep and chill time, to give your body what it needs. Ultimately, I want you to find consistent ways of being active that work for you and complement your life. Initially, you may need to figure out where you can make time for exercise and diarize a few sessions for the week ahead; this is a great way of creating boundaries to engage in self-care practices, which is the ultimate goal of exercise! However, it is worth mentioning here that in pursuit of trying to attain the perfect workout routine, we can fall into the traps of over-training and in some cases exercise addiction.

WHAT IS OVER-TRAINING?

This is when you do too much activity and exercise, which your body then struggles to recover from, resulting in diminished energy and performance. Over-training can be related to frequency of exercise, intensity and lack of rest. The problem with over-training is not only that it often leads to a plateau or decline in training progress, but it can also negatively effect your overall wellbeing. As I explain at the beginning of this book, I myself over-trained for a long time, regularly prioritizing the gym over social occasions and sleep, feeling anxious if I didn't have time to fit in my routine and making my workouts happen no matter what. Exercise became a large part of my identity and a coping mechanism for me, so something that I felt like I *had* to do on many levels. I was definitely over-training and heading down the path to exercise addiction.

HOW TO TELL IF YOU ARE OVER-TRAINING

- » Do you rarely take full rest days (absolutely no exercise)?
- » Do you regularly sacrifice sleep to work out e.g. get up early regardless of what time you went to bed?
- » Have you hit a plateau in training?
- » Do you regularly train until you're exhausted?
- » Is your menstrual cycle affected?

HOW TO TELL IF YOU'RE ADDICTED TO EXERCISE

» Do you feel anxiety about taking rest days?
» Do you feel anxiety or guilt if you don't track ALL your workouts?
» Do you need to burn a certain number of calories per session or hit a certain heart rate?
» Do you prioritize your workouts above other commitments?
» Have your periods stopped?
» Do you continue to exercise despite having injuries?
» Do you spend a lot of time pursuing activities that are related to exercise e.g. highly active holidays?
» Do you feel unable to reduce the amount you exercise despite wanting to?

If you recognize any of the red flags above in yourself and feel that you may have an unhealthy relationship with exercise and/or are regularly over-training, then the best thing to do is to go and see your GP – they can assess your situation and put you in touch with the right healthcare professional so that you can get the help that you deserve. Particularly if your menstrual cycle has been affected, please don't hesitate to seek help.

BUSTING EXERCISE MYTHS

A lot of what we believe about effective workouts and fitness as a whole has largely been influenced by diet culture. So let's look more closely at those beliefs, and bust a few myths.

THE MORE CALORIES BURNT, THE BETTER THE WORKOUT

Nope. A workout that you enjoy and will consistently come back to is best. The focus on burning calories implies that we merely workout to earn and burn food. Quite frankly, that idea needs to die as it can be harmful, not only to our relationship with food, but with exercise too. Go back to the table on page 50 and remember all the other fabulous reasons for moving our bodies. Of course, this myth is broadcast by the many gyms and fitness brands who market their services and products as the ones that will 'burn the most calories', and the growing popularity of fitness trackers and leaderboards in classes is not helping us move away from a calorie focus. I do encourage you to think about switching off the data in order to be more present in mind and body in class. Forget about the calories and focus on how you feel!

IF YOU DIDN'T SWEAT, IT WASN'T A GOOD WORKOUT

Look, some of us are just sweaty people (hello, hi there 🥵), and some of us just aren't. Sweat is our bodies' way of cooling us down. If you regularly work out, then your body's cooling system is likely to kick in quicker than others. But really, it's not a marker of an effective workout. Think about hot yoga – many rave about how great hot yoga is because it makes them sweat. The difference between hot and standard yoga is simply the high temperature of the studio, which causes you to sweat more. If you did exactly the same yoga class in a normal studio and a hot studio, the health benefits would be the same. A hot workout just makes you more dehydrated, so please be sure to drink plenty of water if you sweat.

IF YOU'RE NOT SUPER SORE THE NEXT DAY
THEN YOU DIDN'T WORK HARD ENOUGH

If you're sore the next day, there could me a multitude of reasons for this. The workout may have been challenging on your muscles, which can cause DOMS (delayed onset muscle soreness). How you recover will impact how sore you feel. You should aim to get adequate sleep (7–8 hours a night), eat enough to help muscle recovery before and after your workout (yep, carbs as well as protein and fats). Warming up and cooling down properly and regularly incorporating stretching and mobility into your training also help manage muscle soreness. Doing all of the above should actually help you to avoid feeling like you've been hit by a bus – which isn't the sign of a good workout. The bottom line is, if you aren't sore then it doesn't mean that you haven't gained any benefits from your workout. We're not only moving to challenge our muscles, sometimes the priority of a workout may be getting headspace, having fun with friends or focusing on technique.

YOU NEED TO WORK OUT FOR AT LEAST
AN HOUR FOR IT TO BE EFFECTIVE

Says who? This is another sneaky rule derived from diet culture that stops us from listening to our bodies. If we try to always adhere to it, it's only going to lead to more guilt, shame and feeling like we're not enough when it can't be maintained. But a workout should never make you feel like that... remember we're doing this to feel good! The reality is that we may not always have a full spare hour to commit to exercise. It's not about training for longer, it's about training smarter and using the time you do have to move in a way you enjoy. There is no minimum time requirement, and as you learn to tune into your body through intuitive movement (more on this next), you will learn that some days it's 10 minutes and other days it's 45 minutes and on other occasions you want to go on a long run that takes 2 hours! All are effective and adequate for different reasons.

INTUITIVE MOVEMENT

In the *Eat Happy* section (see page 34), we discussed the concept of intuitive eating as a means to help us cultivate a positive relationship with food and our body. We spoke about the key 10 principles of the concept, as devised by Evelyn Tribole and Elyse Resch in their book *Intuitive Eating*. One of those key principles emphasizes the importance of exercise as joyful movement, which I want to explore further. Because just as we were born intuitive eaters, I believe we were born to think of movement as playtime... but along the way the fun got sucked out. Inspired by the original framework created by Tribole and Resch, I wanted to discuss the ways in which we can rebuild trust with our bodies and find the fun in fitness again.

Registered nutritionist and author of *Just Eat It*, Laura Thomas defines intuitive movement like this:

'Intuitive movement refers to your body's innate ability to communicate how, when, how much, and how often to move. It moves us away from looking at exercising and working out as a means to control our body and towards a way of grounding into and being in our body.'

I see the practice of intuitive movement as a way we can build back up the innate self-trust between ourselves and our bodies. In her book, *The Anatomy of Trust*, research professor Dr. Brené Brown uses the metaphor of a jar of marbles to describe the notion of trust: positive affirmations add marbles in, and moments where the trust is broken gradually take them away. When it comes to trusting our bodies, diet culture and its messaging have given us plenty of reasons to take marbles out of our jar, meaning that some of us are running dangerously low or severely lacking some integral marbles. Listening to advice from 'fitspo' accounts online and copying what they do – despite what your body is feeling – is a marble removed from the jar. Letting a fitness tracker determine how hard you work by focusing on having to hit a certain number of calories per workout deletes another marble. Running because it 'counts' as a workout, even though you hate it and prefer other forms of movement is another marble taken away. So, how can we work on getting more marbles back in your metaphorical jar? Well, it means going on a journey to build trust back up with your body, bit by bit, until we are consistently able to listen to and honour its needs.

To do this, I'm going to take you through how we can draw parallels with the 10 principles of intuitive eating (see page 38 if you need a refresher) and apply them to how we feel about exercise and fitness:

1. REJECT THE DIET MENTALITY – Many of us think of exercise as just a means to just lose weight, which is why all the joy got sucked out of it. It became a chore we had to endure as a means to control our bodies and a way to 'redeem' ourselves after eating certain foods, as prescribed by diet culture. All of this stems from a socially conditioned fear of fatness, and so the aesthetic goals of thinness and leanness have been hugely normalized in modern fitness culture. Deciding to shift the focus of your training to health, enjoyment and performance instead can feel like you're swimming against the tide, so how can we take steps to reject the diet mentality in the context of fitness?

A) RECOGNIZE AND ACKNOWLEDGE THE HARM DIETS DO – Remind yourself that the vast majority of diets are unsuccessful (see page 10) and how they can negatively impact on mental health – when we approach exercise as just part of a diet to manipulate the body, the aim is to see 'results' first and enjoyment and our happiness come last. Then, think about the negative impact that intentional weight loss for aesthetic goals has on body image (see page 23). We also know that dieting is a high-risk factor for developing an eating disorder, and though this is not the case for everyone, it's important to be aware of.

B) BE AWARE OF THE DIET MENTALITY TRAITS AND MINDSET – Be aware of the fitness content that you consume online, in magazines, TV and books etc. – are these resources primarily putting the focus on exercise as a way to 'blast fat' or get you 'visible abs' or a 'bikini body'? Do you consume information from people who are all a similar size with similar backgrounds? I did for a long time, particularly with the fitness accounts I followed on social media. But by filling up my feeds with people of all shapes and sizes, backgrounds and perspectives, I was able to gain a far more balanced view of what different bodies look like in action and take a step back from the diet mentality bubble. Also, be aware of how you feel about taking rest days. Guilt and anxiety about missing a workout or being more sedentary some days are signs that we are still in the diet mentality, with fear of weight gain or changes to our body.

C) GET RID OF THE DIET TOOLS – Many of us have become accustomed to measuring our exercise and fitness success through how defined our abs are or how much we weigh. This makes aesthetics the focus, reinforcing that you are first a body to be looked at, and a person second. This type of measuring cannot quantify your true athletic improvements, which can be measured in so many other ways, such as increases in speed, power and endurance to name just a few (keep reading to learn more about this). So, it's time to get rid of the scales, stop the measurements, take off the fitness trackers and stop taking weekly progress pics. That might feel really overwhelming to do all in one go, so try slowly phasing them out. Aim for one week without, and at the end of the week think about how you feel without these tools. Has it affected how present you are when working out? Have you been looking at your body as much in the mirror? Have your workouts become more or less enjoyable? Have you noticed a difference in motivation or external pressure? It's also important to consider how rigid workout plans and training splits can become a barrier to becoming more in tune with your body and exploring joyful movement. When you feel like you 'have' to follow a plan to the letter, it can lead to guilt or a sense of failure if you struggle to stick to it, much like a diet. If you are still working through your relationship with exercise, put the plan on the back burner, and when you are ready, try one that encourages flexibility, like the one in this book.

D) BE KIND AND COMPASSIONATE TO YOURSELF – Focusing on weight and aesthetics has been the norm in the fitness space for so long, it's likely to feel weird coming at things from a different perspective. Remember, we are all living and swimming in diet culture with a strong current heading in one direction, so you may just need to tread water where you are, take stock of everything and summon up the strength to turn around and head in the opposite direction. We are not bad people for wanting to diet or have weight loss and aesthetic goals. We are human, and we are figuring this stuff out. Shifting from the weight-centric paradigm to a weight-inclusive paradigm will take time, unlearning and bucket loads of compassion along the way.

2. HONOUR YOUR APPETITE FOR EXERCISING + 3. STOP WHEN SATISFIED – We need to work on our awareness of our bodies' appetite for exercise in order to know when it needs more or has had enough and many variables besides. As Laura Thomas' definition of intuitive movement states (see page 57), we need to tune in to our bodies' innate ability to communicate its needs. Think about what it could be trying to tell you:

> » **When do you want to work out – what time of day feels best?**
> » **How long do you want to exercise for?**
> » **What kind of exercise is appealing?**
> » **When is your body telling you 'enough'?**
> » **How energetic do you feel today?**

Listening to your body's answers to the questions above means that you can begin to engage in exercise on your own terms. You can start to explore and find what feels good for you if you're new to exercise, or if you have been stuck in a rut, then stop what you've habitually been doing for a while and try out new ways of doing things. You may want to take a step back from the gym, for example, and instead try hiking outdoors and doing yoga at home. For me, personally, going through this process, I had weight trained with a bodybuilding-style split for years, because it's what I believed was best to manipulate my aesthetics and weight. When the pressure was off and I let myself be free from worrying about those things, my workout horizons hugely expanded. There wasn't a right or wrong way to train anymore, and I wasn't stuck to the rigid confines of what I thought was 'good or bad' when thinking about results. As a personal trainer, I understand the importance of incorporating certain elements in training to build fitness (we will look at this later in this section), but having much more flexibility has meant I have tried new things, challenged my body in new ways and most importantly had fun in the process. Right now, I love spin, weights, reformer Pilates, walking, dance – and I'm hoping to have some swimming lessons too! Now the exercise world is my oyster, and it's yours too! I also encourage this because self-paced exercise that you enjoy doing has been shown to increase likelihood of adherence to regular movement and an improved mood[8, 9]. And we also know that by sticking at something consistently, we will be reaping the health benefits that an active lifestyle brings (see page 50).

4. MAKE PEACE WITH EXERCISE – Perhaps you and exercise have had a rocky all-or-nothing relationship in the past? If you have been a serial dieter and exercise has been a big part of your attempts to lose weight, you may have strong negative associations with slogging your guts out in the gym and tracking each calorie burned. Part of making peace with it is realizing not ALL forms of movement are the same as your bad experience. If you have had negative experiences with a particular form of exercise, it's worth focusing on other ways to get active. See page 53 for inspiration and think about trying other things that might be more fun for you, like a dance class or ice skating. Just as we learned to neutralize food from being 'good' and 'bad' with intuitive eating, we need to do the same with movement, instead recognizing each form of movement has its own merits. There is a little overlap with challenging the fitness police (see next point) here: I have had to unlearn a lot of rules I had around fitness, especially to do with length and frequency of workouts, to make my own peace with it. But now I've got to this place where everything is valid, it's broadened my horizons and given me so many more fun ways to be active.

5. CHALLENGE THE FITNESS POLICE – This is the person, or rather, the little devil on your shoulder, who likes to tell you that yoga isn't a workout, that if you didn't sweat, you didn't work hard enough. It's the voice that says you need to burn a certain number of calories or run a certain distance and that you should be getting a visible result from exercise, or what's the point. This whole process is about dialling down the external noise of the learned rules and regulations around fitness and instead tuning back into the body's wants and needs. When these kinds of policing thoughts arise, push back and challenge them. For example, in a diet mentality you may have told yourself that you should be working out five times a week. However, as you begin to tune into your body, you may find you would like an extra rest day, but as you consider the possibility, feelings of guilt and anxiety pop up. You fear that if you don't work out hard enough your body might change... so question that – what is my body telling me? What are my fears around having an extra rest day? And then challenge those fears by taking the rest day. Each time you rebel against those rules you had in place, you step outside your comfort zone and help to increase its boundaries. Remember that this process is helping *you* become the expert of your body, so start trusting your own judgement.

6. DISCOVER THE FEEL-GOOD FACTOR – Exercise is not a form of punishment. Let me repeat that again... EXERCISE IS NOT A FORM OF PUNISHMENT. I really hope you are learning that contrary to diet culture beliefs, exercise is not about controlling weight, burning calories, earning your next meal and trying to look like a model. Instead, exercise is a form of self-respect, self-care and self-expression. When we consider the physical and mental benefits of exercise, carving out time in your week to move your body is an appointment in your dairy that you should want to look forward to. Maybe that's by making it social – playing a team sport, heading out on a hike with a family member or heading to a dance class with friends? Social connection is a significant factor in contributing to our health and wellbeing, so incorporating it with your exercise means a double whammy to help you feel good.

Furthermore, when you start to be more present in your body and mind during physical activity, you become more aware of all the incredible ways it can make you feel: Perhaps you feel **proud** of hiking up that hill and seeing that incredible view; maybe you felt **strong** when lifting those weights, which gave you a **confidence boost** to take into that tough meeting at work; perhaps it felt **powerful** to punch and kick that bag and let your the frustrations out; maybe you feel a sense of **community and belonging** when playing football with your teammates, or maybe you felt **totally fierce** when nailing that dance routine?

Tip When teaching my classes, I always encourage each participant to reflect on one mini victory they had during the class. We're always pretty quick to focus on the things that we struggled with, being the self-deprecating society that we are, but I invite you to flip that on its head. At the end of each of your workouts, note down at least one little victory, and celebrate all those small wins! You can write this in a journal, or even keep a note on your phone, so eventually you'll have a long list of wins to keep you inspired and motivated.

7. MANAGING EMOTIONS – When life gets tough, exercise can be a helpful coping mechanism and an outlet, but it should not be relied on in place of therapy or professional mental health care. It can only be used as a tool to help support your mental wellbeing when moving from a place of intuition, care and respect. For you, that may be getting outdoors in nature, or putting on boxing gloves and punching stress into a bag. It might include slowing down on sad days and choosing to practice a calming yoga flow. It's about building trust so you can do what's right for your mind and body in the moment as opposed to just 'pushing through' and disregarding how you feel mentally.

8. ACCEPTING YOUR BODY – As we know, diet culture likes to pitch exercise as a way to change your body. The fitness industry loves a before-and-after shot, and so many of us embark on our own journey to try and get the perfect one. But as noted in 'rejecting the diet mentality', we need to push that aside. You don't have to be seeing huge visible results to be benefiting from adding movement into your life. Instead, focus on self-acceptance and body acceptance. Stop punishing your body, stop abusing it, stop comparing it and instead work with it. That is what is at the core of cultivating an intuitive relationship with your body and movement. Even though you've been pitted against each other for so long, you and your body are on the *same team*.

I know that accepting your body can be tough when we live in a society that celebrates thinness and shuns fatness – this isn't necessarily straightforward stuff – however, I hope that the *Get Happy* section of this book (page 14) has given you tools for working towards this. An important part of learning to accept your own body is accepting other people's too. Linda Bacon wrote this brilliant piece on acceptance in her book *Health At Every Size*:

> 'Just as you want others to accept you, it's important that you accept others. While you may be discriminated against because of your body size, others are discriminated against based on their skin colour, ethnic background, sexual orientation, or many other characteristics. Developing open-mindedness and empathy towards others who are discriminated against enables you to support and feel empathy for your own position. Being fat, like being Hispanic or a lesbian, is not bad; it's just different. Our diversity is what makes the world such an exciting place! We can celebrate size diversity in much the same way as we are learning to celebrate cultural diversity.'

As Linda says, body diversity is real! Fit bodies come in all shapes and sizes, as you can see on the cover of this book and by the models used in our training guide. But we don't just want this book to be diverse, we want all our fitness content to be diverse. I thoroughly recommend the following Instagram accounts for more body diversity inspiration:

- » @iamlshauntay
- » @mynameisjessamyn
- » @louisegreen_bigfitgirl
- » @hijabi.lifts
- » @bryonygordon
- » @prettystrongbec
- » @amandalacount
- » @superfithero
- » @sophjbutler
- » @meg.boggs

THINGS TO PRACTICE TO ENCOURAGE BODY ACCEPTANCE:

- » *Appreciate what your body can do* – Celebrate the little wins. Be proud of each small improvement, each increase in strength, stamina, flexibility or co-ordination.
- » *Respect your body* – Joyful movement of any kind is a form of self-care and respect. Exercise is one piece of the puzzle that makes up your health and wellbeing.
- » *Practice self-compassion* – Be kind to yourself through this process. You, your body and your mind are just trying their best to navigate this journey.

9. GENTLE GUIDANCE – This final key principle comes last for good reason. Think of it like this; you know when your favourite necklace turns into a big knot that you struggle to unpick – well that's us to start with, we are the knotted chain. Through each of these intuitive movement principles (and over the course of the book), we've slowly been untangling and unravelling your relationship with exercise (built on the lies of diet culture) so that you can start again with the clear focus you need to tune in with your body's needs. It takes time and work to get to this point; don't underestimate that and don't rush it.

Once you are here (nice and untangled), we can start thinking about adding gentle guidance back into your workouts. This isn't about strict, rigid workout plans, it's about working in the shades of grey. Making sure you are exercising safely and effectively, while giving you the flexibility to follow the structure that is required if you want to meet more performance-related goals. For example, you might choose to work towards running a 10K, signing up for a Tough Mudder or completing your first pull-up – an element of structure and support will be needed to achieve those. Achieving fitness goals can be fun and satisfying – it's cool to see what you and your body are capable of. The difference is, the dieting and all-or-nothing mentality are taken out of the equation.

On page 86, you will find my 10-week Workout Guide. I designed it to help you build a strong physical foundation and let you feel comfortable using weights and performing a range of exercises. I have also tried to keep it flexible and fun, so that you can make it fit in with your lifestyle, your needs and your enjoyment.

RESOLVING FEARS AROUND INTUITIVE MOVEMENT

Some of the ideas discussed here may feel challenging for you, especially if you have had a difficult bond with exercise in the past. Cultivating a healthy and happy relationship with it takes time, work and compassion. It's important to start with 'rejecting the diet mentality', and then work through the remaining key principles, leaving 'gentle guidance' until the end. It may not be a straight path, and you may well identify sticking points that require more attention. Below, I've attempted to anticipate and respond to any fears you might have about fully leaning in to this process:

FEAR: *If I stop a structured plan and just listen my body, I won't do anything at all*
REALITY: There may be moments of working through this process when you *don't* do anything, and that's okay. The pendulum needs to swing one way and then the other in order to recalibrate and find your sweet spot somewhere in the middle. If exercise has been strongly associated with body transformation for you, then taking this out of the equation might leave you've lost motivation briefly. But just go back and remind yourself of the incredible benefits of movement (see page 50) and start thinking about, and even writing down, how they could fit into the context of your life.

FEAR: *But If I change the way I move and work out, then my body will change*
REALITY: Yes, it might, but if you're happier enjoying the way you move your body, feeling less guilt and anxiety around exercise and still reaping the health benefits that come with regular movement, then isn't it worth it? Isn't the freedom and fun that come with intuitive and joyful movement worth celebrating more than a dress size? It's normal to fear change in appearance, particularly weight gain, as we live in a society that demonizes fatness. Part of this process is challenging that and trying to let go of that pressure as you learn to have fun with movement again. If this fear resonates with you, turn back to page 10 where Laura Thomas explains why diets don't work.

FEAR: *If I work out intuitively without the same rigid structure, then I won't be able to achieve my goals of getting fitter or stronger as my training won't be as consistent*
REALITY: As you are discovering how to intuitively exercise, you will need to hit pause on performance goals initially because they will stand in the way of building intuition with your body. Training may feel more sporadic and less intentional, but exploring structure vs no structure and what works for you as an individual is part of the process. That's not to say you can't ever have performance goals again, (I actively encourage them on page 76) but it's important to remove the boundaries at first to give you clarification on what your real motivation is and the freedom to explore what feels good. Whether you are usually driven by goals or not, there may still be times in our lives when we take a break to move our bodies just for the enjoyment in the moment.

A NOTE ON FITNESS TRACKERS + DEVICES

Intuitive movement is all about taking external influences out of the equation and working on strengthening the connection between you and your body. Because of this, I think it's important to explore the role of increasingly common fitness trackers and devices in more depth. They may seem your best friend at first, but there are a few reasons why I think they can be a barrier to building trust with your body:

1. During a workout itself they can be distracting and hold you back from being truly present. I was teaching a class on a retreat recently where one of the participants kept tapping their watch between every exercise, or sometimes even during the actual movement, to see how high their heart rate was and how many calories were being burned. Ironically, because of this interference, they weren't able to move to the full intensity of what they were truly capable of. For the next session, I asked if they might experiment trying a class without the watch. The next day, this person was noticeably more present, focused and determined to give the class full energy and enjoyment.

2. They can contribute to the guilt, shame and anxiety around exercise if we don't burn a certain number of calories or stay in a certain heart rate zone for long enough. In the past, I've done a really fun workout, challenged myself and then looked at my fitness tracker, only for it to make me feel like what I did was inadequate. Also the 'doesn't count unless I tracked it' mentality isn't benefiting anyone.

3. Daily step goals, movement goals and calorie targets don't understand your life. The amount we move from one day to the next will naturally fluctuate as life does. Sometimes we are going to have more sedentary days and at other times highly active ones. The additional pressure of having to hit a certain static goal every day is unnecessary. I advocate being active whenever possible, but having a set goal that is the same each day is not realistic.

In conclusion, I challenge you to have a go at moving your body without tracking it, without knowing how many calories you've burned and without knowing how many steps you've done or which heart rate zone you were in. I believe that it's the only way to get back to your body and your own internal device.

MY EXERCISE GUIDELINES

Once you have worked through the principles of intuitive movement and feel in a good place with your relationship with fitness, we can start re-introducing moderate structure following the gentle guidance principle. In this section, I'm going to give you the knowledge and understanding you need to navigate your own path in a fitness environment, by teaching you about the different types of training and their benefits.

WEIGHT TRAINING

Also known as resistance training or strength training. There are some variables, but essentially this type of training involves bearing weight through lifting or moving weights, and/or your own bodyweight. The NHS recommends resistance training twice a week to reap the benefits of the full list below, but even one session a week has positive effects in the following areas:

- » positive effects on the musculoskeletal system
- » increases in bone density (which helps prevent osteoporosis)
- » increases in everyday functional strength
- » helps reduce lower back pain
- » helps reduce sarcopenia (loss of body mass)
- » improves posture
- » increases metabolic rate

Resistance training does not necessarily require the use of heavy weights, but should involve precise, controlled movements for each major muscle group. Exercises that target more than one major muscle group are called compound movements – I like to think of these as just getting more bang for your buck. For example, a weight-bearing squat is a compound move because it will mainly focus on quadriceps, glutes and calves, but also engage the muscles in the core and back if bearing weight. The opposite to this is isolation movements, which only work one muscle at a time.

KEY COMPOUND MOVEMENTS

Squat variations back squats, goblet squats, box squats, single leg squats, step-ups, lunges etc. These predominantly focus on the muscles in your legs, so quadriceps, glutes and calves.

Hinge variations deadlifts, romanian deadlifts, stiff leg deadlifts, kettlebell swings, good mornings, rack pulls, hip thrusts etc. These predominantly focus on the posterior chain, which is made up of hamstrings, glutes and *erector spinae* a.k.a. the lower back, buttocks and backs of your legs.

Push variations chest press, bench press, push-ups, shoulder press, tricep dips etc. These exercises target the pectorals, deltoids, biceps and triceps, a.k.a. the chest, shoulders and arms.

Pull variations pull-ups, chin-ups, barbell and dumbbell rows, single arm rows, lat-pull downs etc. These exercises are targeting the main muscles in your back; _latisimus dorsi,_ _trapezius_ and rear deltoids.

Core/loaded carries plank variations, deadbugs, farmer walks, pallof press etc. These focus on the core; transverse abdominals, which brace the core like a corset around our waist, as well as obliques and rectus abdominals.

KEY ISOLATION MOVEMENTS
These are the extra things you may want to do towards the end of a workout if you want to work on building strength in a specific area, for example bicep curls, tricep extensions and calf raises.

TYPES OF WEIGHT TRAINING
ENDURANCE
Rep range: 13–20+
Rest time between sets: 30–60 seconds
This is the low-weight, high-rep style of training that you are likely to come across in a class-based environment such as body pump. This type of weight training is the perfect introduction for many beginners, but also a great way to train for endurance-related activities like long-distance running.

HYPERTROPHY
Rep range: 7–12
Rest time between sets: 30–60 seconds
The aim with hypertrophy training is to increase muscle fibres, which therefore increases overall muscle mass and thus strength too. The most effective exercises for this are ones that contract the muscle against resistance repeatedly. Body builders and regular gym-goers who are very focused on building muscle strength are likely to work in this area.

STRENGTH
Rep range: 0–6
Rest time between sets: 3–5 minutes
The aim here is to build muscle and increase strength by working with maximum effort on compound movements. Think power lifters and those who #liftheavy.

WEIGHT-TRAINING EQUIPMENT

There is such a variety of ways to lift and move weight and I encourage you to make use of that fact to keep your training fun and interesting. The table below offers ideas for different types of weights, tools and machines you can use.

FREE WEIGHTS	EXTRAS/BODYWEIGHT TOOLS	MACHINES
» Barbells	» TRX (suspension training)	» Leg press
» Dumbbells	» Sliders	» Chest press
» Kettlebells	» Resistance bands	» Cable machines
» Sandbells	» Small-looped resistance bands	» Lat pulldown machine
» Weight plates		» Leg curl/hamstring curl
» Medicine balls	» Swiss ball	» Shoulder press
» ViPR (cylinder with handles)	» Ab wheel	» Smith machine
» Sled	» BOSU (balance trainer)	» Hack squat
» Tyre	» Box	» Assisted pull-up machine
» Battle ropes	» Olympic rings	» Seated row machine

BODYWEIGHT TRAINING

This form of weight training involves using your own body weight to create resistance. It's great if you like to work out outside, at home or if you travel a lot, as you can do it in virtually any space, at any time. It's also free!

Bodyweight training is a great place to start if you're new to weights. For example, it's always best to nail a bodyweight squat before adding weights to the mix to build up a base level of strength. However, some of the key compound movements in resistance training, as previously discussed, are bodyweight-based – pull-ups being a great example. You can also incorporate bodyweight training into other forms of training, for instance, you will see in the training guide (see page 86) that the resistance workouts are a hybrid of weight-bearing exercises and bodyweight exercises such as press-ups and plank variations.

You might hear some people refer to bodyweight training as calisthenics. This is the combination of bodyweight strength training combined with gymnastics to produce moves such as handstands, human flags and muscle-ups. It focuses on mobility, flexibility, strength and, most importantly, play to learn new skills while having fun in the process.

CARDIOVASCULAR TRAINING

You most likely know this as cardio. As with weight training, I would recommend that everyone regularly incorporates some form of cardio-based exercise into their routine. In fact, NHS guidelines recommend 150 minutes of moderately intense physical activity a week, or 75 minutes of vigorous aerobic activity. Any exercise that increases your heart rate and blood circulation throughout the body counts as cardio – so you can get creative with how you choose to move!

Like any muscle, your heart benefits from being worked, and regular cardio can improve strength and overall heart health. It is also a great way to increase the production of endorphins, which help produce positive feelings and lessen perception of pain. As we said back on page 19, it also supports your mental health by helping reduce and manage symptoms of anxiety and depression.

STEADY STATE CARDIO

This is low intensity, long duration exercise where you would typically be training at 40–60% of your maximum heart rate and for at least 40 minutes. You may have also heard people refer to LISS training, which stands for Low Intensity Steady State training; forms of this may include cycling, jogging, brisk walking or dancing. This is the least demanding form of cardio and a great place to start if you're new to it. While you're doing it, you should be able to hold a conversation with a 4–6 (low-to-medium) on the RPE scale (rate of perceived exertion).

MEDIUM INTENSITY CARDIO

This is working at a medium level of intensity for a medium amount of time. You would typically be working at 70% of your maximum heart rate for anywhere between 20–60 minutes. This may include more intense cycling, running, rowing or swimming etc. Your rate of perceived exertion should be about a 7–8 on the RPE scale, where breathing becomes heavier and it's harder to chat.

HIGH INTENSITY INTERVAL TRAINING

A popular form of training, more commonly known as HIIT. It is aerobic training with the aim of working at upwards of 80–90% of your maximum heart rate. Working intervals, which are strenuous to complete, can range from 60 to 240 seconds, followed by periods of rest lasting a similar time period. For example, 1 minute of intense running followed by 1 minute of walking. HIIT sessions will last between 5–20 minutes and should be no longer if you are working at maximum effort. The rate of perceived exertion is 8–9 on the scale, and so you should feel fatigued after completing the workout and struggle to talk. When completed at full capacity, this form of training is tough on your central nervous system so you should allow at least 48 hours to recover afterwards.

FARTLEK TRAINING

Meaning 'speed play' in Swedish, this type of training originated in Sweden. It is an opportunity to have fun and do a mixture of all the different types of cardio mentioned previously. You might like to do a 10-minute run, directly followed by a 2-minute walk, finishing with a 1-minute sprint etc. This particular protocol complements intuitive movement well, as you can dictate how fast, slow and how long you want to move.

CIRCUIT TRAINING/CONDITIONING

This can include a mix of weight-based exercises, such as walking lunges, combined with more traditional cardio-based exercises, such as skipping. A circuit might feature eight exercises to be completed in intervals of 40 seconds at each station, with 20 seconds rest in between. It's a great way to keep it varied and include a variety of exercises that challenge the whole body. Depending on exercise selection and your fitness levels, the heart rate level will vary, but should generally be between 4–9 on the RPE scale.

BALANCE + FLEXIBILITY TRAINING

The incorporation of balance and flexibility into a workout routine is often overlooked. Obvious examples of this type of exercise include yoga, Pilates, barre and tai chi. We put so much emphasis on exerting force with our muscles through weights and raising our heart rate with cardio, but we also need to prioritize connecting with our bodies through movement. Not only does this type of training help to keep you more mobile and supple in everyday life, it complements other forms of training through giving a greater range of motion, which can aid strength and fitness and reduce risk of injury.

YOGA

I asked expert yoga teacher Jonelle Lewis to tell us a little bit more about the different forms of yoga and its physical and mental health benefits.

WHAT IS YOGA?

There are a lot of different definitions of yoga. One often put forward is the definition, 'union'. A union of what? A union of you... all the parts of you... making up a whole and integrated being. Yoga is a psycho-spiritual practice developed in Northern India over 4000 years ago. It made its way to the West around the 1930s and, since then, millions of people have started adding it to their self-care regimes. Yoga isn't all about trying to do handstands or fancy poses, instead it's a tool for living and a way of connecting to our highest self. It's a practice that helps to unlock our potential; a practice that helps us to manage our lives; a practice that connects us to ourselves.

WHY YOGA?

The benefits of yoga and meditation go way beyond the physical. It's true that practicing certain types of modern postural yoga can get you fit and flexible physically, but yoga's most potent benefit is what it does for the mind and nervous system: it helps manage stress, anxiety and depression and can help with getting better and more restful sleep. It helps to boost the immune system and has been shown to improve body image.

WHAT IS THE ENTRY POINT TO YOGA?

Most of us in the West enter yoga through 'asana' postural yoga, the physical side of the yoga practice. There are many styles, forms and schools of asana yoga. Below, I've listed some of the main types we see in studios and gyms and categorized them further based on the physical effort involved.

LOW IMPACT

MEDITATION

Meditation is at the heart of all yoga practice. One of the reasons we do physical asana practice is to be able to sit quietly without too many distractions from the body. There are many forms of meditation – mostly it is done seated, but it can also be practiced standing, walking and lying down. In meditation, the main focuses are being present, connecting to the self, turning inwards, awareness, mindfulness and stillness. Meditation is not the opposite of thinking, but you might be encouraged to focus on your breath or on one point of concentration. Everyone can benefit from a meditation practice.

RESTORATIVE

This type of yoga is designed specifically for us overworked, overstimulated, overtired, overstressed Westerners! This practice focuses on relaxation for the nervous system. Poses are mostly done lying down and supported over bolsters using props such as straps, blocks, eye-bags and blankets.

YIN

Yin yoga requires the muscles to be relaxed instead of engaged. Poses are passive and held for 2–5 minutes with the option to use props as support. The purpose is to work into the connective tissue (fascia) and load the ligaments in a safe way. While there isn't a lot of movement, the practice brings a lot of sensation and helps with mindfulness and awareness.

MEDIUM IMPACT

HATHA

The general definition of yoga practice, this combines physical poses, breathing techniques and meditation. Most hatha classes encourage use of props. They are a great place to start for beginner yogis as they tend to be slower paced.

LYENGAR

This practice uses a detailed structural approach and is a great way to learn the fundamentals of yoga postures. Props are often used to enable students to feel the benefits of a whole range of postures and everyone is encouraged to progress at their own pace.

KUNDALINI

This type of yoga focuses on mantra, pranayama, mudra, meditation and rhythmic/static asana to target the glandular system and central nervous system to balance the body. This yoga is designed to help balance the inner workings of the body and to build mental stamina.

HIGH IMPACT

ASHTANGA

A physically demanding practice which serves as a workout. Poses are held for five breaths and practiced in a set sequence. Most classes taught are Primary Series (meaning there are six sequences). Ashtanga has a flowing style, which most vinyasa classes are influenced by.

BIKRAM/HOT

Here, a sequence of postures and breathing exercises is done in a studio heated to 32-40 degrees celsius. The intention is that the warmth means muscles are more flexible. Some hot classes are more static coming in and out of postures, others are more flowing vinyasa style.

DYNAMIC/POWER

A more fitness-based way of practicing vinyasa yoga. It is flowing and poses are not held for long.

VINYASA

More of a dynamic style of yoga where breath and movement are linked. Postures are held for a relatively short time and transition from pose to pose is as important as the poses themselves. This practice develops strength and stamina, as well as fluid and graceful movement.

On different days we need different things, so hopefully the groupings and descriptions above will assist you in picking the practice that will be suitable for you physically, mentally and emotionally. As well as supporting all other types of physical activity, the mental and emotional stability that yoga gives can help in every aspect of our lives. There will be a style or practice suitable for you, no matter your gender, age or body type. The best thing is, yoga is for everybody!

PILATES

Another wonderful form of balance and flexibility training, I asked Pilates expert and fitness trainer Hollie Grant to tell us more about Pilates and its benefits.

Often confused with yoga or simply avoided for fear of it being boring, Pilates is anything but! Pilates is a low-impact form of exercise that aims to strengthen the body, increase flexibility, reduce muscle imbalances and, in turn, improve posture. It is a safe, but effective, form of exercise and therefore can be adapted for those who are pre-or post-natal or injured. It's commonly recommended by doctors and physiotherapists for those with back pain, but it is equally effective for those who simply seek ultimate, and functional, bad-ass strength.

Originally named 'Contrology', Pilates was created almost 100 years ago by Joseph Pilates (yes, he was an actual person). Its initial purpose was to assist dancers with their strength, flexibility and range of movement, thus preventing them from injury. Joseph himself was a sickly child who, as a teen, developed a thirst for knowledge for physical strength and anatomy. He went on to become a professional gymnast, boxer and circus performer until World War 1 when he was interned, along with fellow German citizens. This was when he began to train fellow prisoners and evolve his teaching methods. Once released he continued developing this method, collaborating with dance experts such as Rudolf Laban, before finally emigrating to New York and opening a studio with his wife Clara. As we have learned more about physiology in the last 100 years, Pilates has developed and has become more dynamic. However, many instructors still teach the exact repertoire Joseph used, known as 'Classical Pilates'.

The focus in Pilates is core strength. As instructors, we believe the abdominals (and surrounding muscles) act as your powerhouse, and postural issues often stem from a weak core. You'll also find we talk a lot about anatomy and technique in Pilates; it's an educational type of training where those taking part will learn a lot about their bodies. Personally, one of my favourite aspects of Pilates is its focus on the 'mind-body connection'. This requires you to tune in to exactly what you are feeling during each exercise, rather than allowing the mind to aimlessly wander. Many people, including myself, find this helps them to 'switch off' from their worries and concerns and gives them valuable headspace.

There are various different ways to undertake Pilates. It is most commonly mat-based and requires little to no equipment. However, there are various specific apparatus, such as the Reformer, Cadillac or Wunda Chair and these are usually found in more specialist studios. Similarly, how you can practice Pilates varies; it can be practiced in a group or on a one-to-one basis, whereby you are led through a sequence of exercises by your instructor.

One common myth with Pilates is that it is easy – but please don't be fooled (I'd happily show you otherwise). Pilates will help you find muscles you didn't even know existed and will give you the strongest, most functional body you've ever had. So, go and find your nearest studio and you'll never look back!

CROSS-TRAINING

By discussing the various ways to exercise, I have been inadvertently introducing you to the idea of cross-training. This means incorporating a variety of different training methods that complement and support your overarching goals. For example, a runner training for a marathon will greatly benefit from including a mixture of strength, cardio, balance and flexibility-based activities into their workout schedule, as this will help improve performance and prevent injury.

So, incorporating these types of exercise, in the context of a workout week for the 'average' person might look like this:

- » **Monday: weight-based workout**
- » **Tuesday: swimming**
- » **Wednesday: rest**
- » **Thursday: gym class (weights based)**
- » **Friday: yoga**
- » **Saturday: long walk**
- » **Sunday: rest**

There is so much variety and so much to choose from when it comes to fitness, so you can tailor a week of workouts that suits you perfectly. There are no hard and fast rules, it's just about being mindful of how you may benefit from certain categories of exercise (which I've explained in this section), and therefore finding your favourite way to move within that category. I would recommend including some of the following types of session in your cross-training each week for general fitness. Below are some ideas of what this may look like, but feel free to get creative.

1–2 resistance sessions a week
 weight training, weights-based classes, suspension training, bodyweight resistance training, CrossFit etc.

1–2 cardio sessions a week
running, swimming, cycling, dancing, hiking, interval training etc.

1-2 balance, flexibility and mobility sessions a week
yoga, Pilates, barre, tai chi etc.

TRACKING PROGRESS

Traditionally, diet culture has told us to track progress by stepping on the scales, testing body fat percentages, taking measurements and progress pictures. But this constantly reinforces the idea that exercise is not valid unless you are losing weight and transforming your appearance. This is how a lot of the fitness industry operates; in a weight-centric paradigm that considers 'results' to be weight loss and fat loss. But we know it's about so much more than that! You CAN have improvements in fitness, strength, balance and flexibility without the number on the scales changing. What I find most frustrating is that often progress in strength, endurance and stamina is overlooked, because the number of inches or weight lost seems to bear greater value. A person may have gone from being able to do 0 press-ups to being able to complete 5 full bodyweight press-ups, and yet if their weight stays the same, to them it might still feel like a failure?! In my eyes, that improvement in strength is the real achievement to be proud of and celebrated. I believe in actually tracking what matters: the physical, tangible progress AND the overall happiness, confidence and wellbeing of each individual. Here are three weight-neutral ways of tracking progress:

1. Log workouts I choose to log all my PT clients' workouts into a book where we write down the exercise completed, the weight used and how many reps. It's pretty simple, but week on week we aim to progress the programmed exercises by increasing weight or rep count. This means we can track progress in strength and each new PB (of any exercise) is celebrated with a high five and a star in the book! The log books belong to my clients, so they can update them when they're not with me too, and look back to see how far they've come.

2. Take fitness assessments This can include a series of exercises that get tested every 4–8 weeks depending on the programming. For example, a generic test may include number of press-ups to failure, timed full plank to failure, timed wall-sit until failure and how long it takes to row 500 metres. In the case of the workout guide included in this book, I have included a personal best test at weeks 5 and 10, where you perform the same chosen exercise and aim to improve or match your PB. My hope is that by the end, you realize how far you have come and celebrate your improvement, no matter how big or small.

3. Keep a mood diary As you start your training, note how you feel in your body, in your mind and in spirit. Perhaps that may be noting how you feel before and after an individual workout. Or maybe it's journalling about how increases in fitness and strength over time have positively impacted your confidence and self-esteem. It's just as important to be aware of improvements in happiness and wellbeing, as that is what this is truly all about.

FITNESS GOALS

So far, we have discussed all the benefits of working out, and how we can use those to motivate us to move more, but let's look more specifically into the types of goals we can choose to have in the context of weight-inclusive fitness:

STRENGTH this could be increasing bodyweight strength, for example, completing full press-ups, holding a plank or completing a full pull-up etc. It could also be increasing the amount of weight lifted and/or the number of repetitions for any resistance-based exercise.

ENDURANCE within your chosen discipline such as running, rowing, swimming, cycling or hiking etc. see how far you can cover in distance. You could also take into account how long you can maintain a certain pace for over a set distance.

SPEED how quickly can you do something within your chosen discipline – sprint 200 metres? Or row 400 metres? You can also combine speed with strength to focus on power as a fitness goal, and you could think of this in the context of plyometrics, for example, measuring how high or far can you jump?

BALANCE you can focus on improving balance in practices such as yoga, with a focus on how long you can hold challenging poses for.

FLEXIBILITY working on lengthening muscles and improving mobility will increase your flexibility. You may notice improvements in everyday functional movements, or with exercises such as overhead squats, deadlifts or the ability to reach new levels in disciplines such as yoga or Pilates.

MOBILITY increased range of motion is most noticeable in areas such as the ankles, hips, back and shoulders. You can aim for things like increased depth of squats and ease of movement in shoulder press exercises, for example.

COORDINATION this is often sport specific. Think about improving agility and reflexes to become better at your chosen sport, for example, tennis or netball.

JOY this one doesn't have a specific target to reach or an event to prepare for, but is an ongoing thing you can feel.

But, plot twist *YOU DON'T HAVE TO HAVE A SPECIFIC GOAL IF YOU DON'T WANT ONE.*

I'm well aware that some people thrive off of working towards specific goals and tracking progress, and others just enjoy moving their body because it makes them feel good. At different points in our lives we might have specific goals for personal reasons, such as raising money for a charity or cause close to your heart by training for and running a marathon. But by practicing intuitive movement, we can work with our bodies and decide what's best for ourselves as each new year comes and goes.

REST + RECOVERY

I want to make this really clear: **rest is just as important as exercise!**

Rest encompasses taking enough days off from training and prioritizing sleep. Including adequate periods of rest in your training is important because this is when (to put it in a very non-science-y way) 'the magic happens'. What that really means is that your body has the opportunity to process your workouts and adapt to the stress it has been through. Working out (especially weight training) causes the muscle fibres to get micro-tears. When the body rests, it repairs them and at the same time grows more muscle fibres. Without sufficient time to do this, the body will continue to break down muscle tissue from intensive exercise (rather than make more), and we need our muscle tissue as that's the good stuff! Replenishing glycogen stores through food and hydration is also an important part of the reparation process. A good way to motivate yourself to have more rest days is to think of yourself as an athlete, whose aim it is to maintain optimal performance and function.

SLEEP

As my mum has ALWAYS said whenever I've felt overwhelmed, run down or fatigued... 'you just need a good night's sleep'. Turns out, she was right! In his book *Why We Sleep*, Professor Matthew Walker states that 'sleep is the foundation of good health', going on to say that 'most of us do not realize how remarkable a panacea sleep truly is'[10].

Sleep deprivation (6 hours or less a night) is linked to increased risk of disease, poor general health and mental health. It is also linked to poor sporting performance and increased risk of injury. You might think that cutting short your eight hours of sleep to fit in a workout is a sensible thing to do, but research suggests that a full eight hours of sleep is more important than a workout, and that by skipping the last two hours, you not only increase health risks, but physical performance will be worsened. When it's lacking adequate sleep, the body is quicker to fatigue, has less sustained strength and aerobic output can be significantly reduced – not great for working towards your fitness goals. In fact, with each hour of sleep lost, the risk of injury becomes greater[11], so by giving your body ample time to recover from and process your training, you can get the most out of your workouts. In his book, Walker describes sleep as the best legal performance-enhancing drug and he actually advises professional sports teams on how good-quality sleep before and after games/matches can have a hugely positive effect on performance.

It works the other way around too, and exercise can play a great role in helping you sleep better by expending energy in the day. But note that it is best to stop exercising 2–3 hours before bedtime to give yourself time to wind down.

INJURIES

There's no denying it, injuries suck! Which is why many people decide to ignore them and try to soldier on despite their body screaming at them to slow down. But acknowledging and respecting your injuries is another important part of cultivating intuition and trust with your body. As the old adage says, 'it's a short-term sacrifice for a long-term gain'. If we don't give our body the time it needs to completely recover, we risk being susceptible to more injuries further down the road. It's also important to stress that good physiotherapists, sports masseuses and osteopaths are worth the investment, and can work wonders helping to manage and rehabilitate injuries.

As well as the physical, it is important to think about the impact of an injury on our mental health too. I know it's tough to take time out, when with this often comes feelings of frustration at loss of progress or – what I hear most commonly – fear of weight gain. It's totally normal to feel uncomfortable about your body changing, but I hope I've busted enough myths surrounding diet culture at this point in the book to give you some support in that area. So just remember how smart your body is and try to work with it in order to heal it and honour its needs. Whether you're out of the game for one week out or even a whole year, this time is just a drop in the ocean of your whole life. There is no deadline on engaging in joyful movement, so just think of the bigger picture as you embark on your recovery.

ILLNESS

Similarly to injuries, it isn't worth exacerbating ill health symptoms for the sake of working out. As you continue to build attunement with your body, awareness of how it feels to be on top form and how it feels to be functioning below par increases. So, listen to your body, and be sure to recharge your metaphorical batteries until they're back at 100% through rest, sleep and relaxation before getting moving again. This may mean taking some full rest days so you can get back to full capacity more quickly, or adapting training to focus more on low intensity work such as a gentle yoga class or walk to aid recovery. 'Short-term loss for long-term gain' is most definitely the mantra to remember!

CONFIDENCE IN A FITNESS ENVIRONMENT

Due to lack of body and ethnic diversity, sadly the fitness world can be an intimidating and/or unwelcoming place. It would have you believe that gyms are solely populated with models, body builders and those with a single digit body fat percentage, as that is how mainstream fitness markets itself. I would hate for that to hold anyone back from going to classes or working out in a gym-type environment if that's what they would like to do. So, below I've aimed to shed some light on the reality of working out in a fitness space or at the gym.

BELIEF: *I'm not fit enough*
REALITY: There is no pre-requisite fitness level needed to join a class or go to a gym. No matter your fitness level, we are all equally entitled to be there. In fact, I would argue that regular gym goers should be extra accommodating towards those starting out. As a personal trainer, I love working with beginners, as we can build good habits and a strong foundation straight out of the gate.

BELIEF: *The weights section is only for men*
REALITY: The weights area of any gym can be intimidating if it's populated by more men than women. However, the number of women taking interest in the weights area has increased hugely in the last five years, so you might be surprised to see more women there than you'd think. Once again, if you don't want to talk to anyone or make eye contact with them, listen to a podcast or put on your favourite playlist and focus on what YOU are doing, and how good your workout makes you feel.

BELIEF: *I'm scared to try something new for fear of judgement*
REALITY: If we never tried anything new in life, we wouldn't ever make progress. There is a lot to be said for expanding the boundaries of your comfort zone. We have all been beginners! If you don't know where to start with a particular exercise, google it. If you need help with executing, ask a team member of the gym to help. Or even better, use the workout guide at the back of the book and look up the accompanying videos!

BELIEF: *The gym is full of people who look like #fitspos and I won't fit in*
REALITY: I'm not saying that there won't be people who look like #fitspos at the gym, but they will be in the minority. Because in real life, there are few people with those genetics. However, because of societal beauty standards, they get given the greatest platforms due to their privilege. We are shown a skewed version of what fit people look like, and we think they only look one way – but body diversity is real! Just take a look at the women featured in this book.

THE FITNESS INDUSTRY
+ DIET CULTURE

I hope that by this point in the book you are starting to get a clear idea of how diet culture has pervaded the fitness industry, our relationships with food, exercise and our own body image (see diet culture definition on page 9 if you need a refresher). However, diet culture likes to be sneaky, it's a bit like a shape shifter, showing up under different guises, so next I want to explore how the fitness industry enforces diet culture in greater depth.

BEFORE AND AFTER PHOTOS + BODY TRANSFORMATIONS

You know the classic 12-week (or any timeframe, really) before and after photos – bigger body on the left with relaxed posture, the person looks sad and disheveled. Then on the right you have a smiley, shiny, tanned, smaller body, shown posing and flexing muscles. The implication is that anyone with the body on the left shouldn't accept themselves as they are. These photos are saying that people are altogether better when they are leaner and smaller, which plays into our culture of fat phobia. So, what message does this send to those whose body may be bigger than the 'before' photo? It says there is something wrong with this body type, that needs to be fixed. It evokes feelings of shame and guilt that no one should ever be made to feel with regards to their body.

Now, we know that this form of marketing is all about showing how effective a certain plan or style of training is. Some of the biggest names in the fitness industry have built online empires off the back of these before and after images. But I have met many clients who have not had their desired result from doing these online plans. It's important to consider how many people have purchased these apps and plans, versus how many have actually achieved their weight loss goal and maintained it long term. A study was completed on how effective diet books are in comparison to their Amazon reviews[12]. People who had lost a big amount of weight and had 'successful' results left glowing reviews on Amazon recommending everyone buy the book because it worked for them. However, the reality of how much most people lost on these diets can be seen in the graph on the right. With the Amazon review (black) reporting far greater weight loss than the research (green, blue, brown).

If we compare this evidence to the before and after photos shared by fitness gurus on social media, the truth is that only a small minority of people achieve and sustain those dramatic results, but many more invest in the same plan and yet don't experience the same outcome. Diet culture makes you think you've failed if you don't get 'results', but as we've learned, the majority of diets are not sustainable long term, and our bodies are wired to resist.

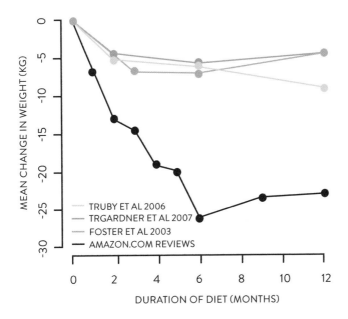

TRUBY ET AL 2006
TRGARDNER ET AL 2007
FOSTER ET AL 2003
AMAZON.COM REVIEWS

MEAN CHANGE IN WEIGHT (KG)

DURATION OF DIET (MONTHS)

Sharing inspiring body transformation stories has also become the marketing go-to for gyms and personal trainers. It is widely encouraged as part of a successful business strategy, and you can even go on courses to learn how. But this just perpetuates the idea that exercise and training are only about weight loss and aesthetics, and training to get those before and after type 'results'.

Personal trainers have in the past challenged my views on this by arguing 'clients come to me asking for weight loss, wanting the after photo. Who am I to deny them?' My response: 'clients have come to you with those requests because that is what you have marketed to them'. The marketing has shamed them into believing that completing a body transformation will make them happy. But what the photos fail to show is what usually happens after those 12 weeks. When biology kicks in and fights back at the intentional weight loss by making it harder to maintain and sustain the methods that got them there in the first place. What's not shown is what happens if and when they gain weight back. Will they then go to more extreme lengths to get back to that original after photo? How is their relationship with food and exercise? Has it impacted their social life and relationships?' These are the types of questions we need answers to.

Personally, I have never used this strategy for my own personal training business, as even before I discovered the weight-inclusive approach, it just didn't sit right with me. However, I have used before and after pictures of *myself* on social media as a form of marketing to help build my online presence. It's always been interesting to me that these types of images and posts received the most engagement. They only reinforced my own self-objectification and communicated that I was a body first and a person second. I'll be honest and say, it's pretty addictive when people are praising you, but this ultimately just fuelled my disordered relationship with food and fitness. I do now regret my choice to share those, as I feel it has only contributed to weight stigma, fat phobia and diet culture's narrative that fit and healthy looks a certain way.

NOT A DIET, A LIFESTYLE CHANGE
One of the ways diet culture creeps in is when it's described as a 'lifestyle change'. So you may not be on a formal diet with strict protocol BUT you may still be cutting certain foods out, restricting intake or exercising in a certain way motivated by weight loss or fat loss. Even though I would never have admitted to being on a diet at the time, I mentioned at the beginning of the book that I worked with a nutritionist and a personal trainer two years ago in order to lose some weight and 'lean up' for the summer. I felt uncomfortable with my weight gain, as I had internalized that this was wrong, and had been looking for a way to control that. I knew I didn't want to diet again but I was still in a restrictive mindset, hoping for a change in aesthetics to use as a marker of success.

CUTTING + BULKING
This is a form of dieting is focused on fat loss (cutting) and building muscle through eating in a surplus (bulking). Extreme examples of this are body building, bikini and fitness competitions. Traditionally, you may have heard #fitspos talk about bulking through winter to build muscle, and then in spring/summer dieting or cutting to 'reveal' all of the hard work. All of this is usually done through tracking macros, which dictates how much protein, carbohydrates and fat you should eat combined with a structured training plan. Like any form of dieting, this comes with the potential to binge after a period of restriction, commonly known as a 'cheat day'. This form of dieting and training is really good at ignoring the body's intuition, as it's very much about following strict external rules. When I first started my fitness journey, this was my diet of choice and everything became a numbers game. My connection with internal cues had been completely cut – at times I was left hungry but with no macros left I wasn't allowed to eat, and at other times I was eating way past fullness to hit my daily numbers. It was the opposite of intuitive eating and intuitive movement.

BIKINI BODY WORKOUT
Similar names for this include: little black dress workout, beach body or summer body, lean body workout etc. When the name implies you have to conform to a certain beauty standard or body ideal then, yep, you guessed it... it's diet culture. These terms are really popular on social media, with many communities built through participating together and sharing how much weight is visibly lost.

NAVIGATING DIET CULTURE IN A FITNESS ENVIRONMENT

Now we know what to look out for, how do we protect ourselves from diet culture rearing its ugly head in a fitness space? This may turn up as conversations in the changing rooms, in the choice of language used by an instructor, or in a one-to-one situation with a trainer. Perhaps you see or hear things that don't sit right with you or make you feel self-conscious.

In Australia, a study by Leah Gilbert's Body Positive Athletes found that 85% of respondents said that having a body positive, weight-neutral environment was hugely important to long-term participation in physical activity. So, what can we do about this? Well, the power actually lies with you, the consumer, the client. Your feedback, whether anonymous or not, is effective. If we want to collectively change the narrative within fitness and push the industry towards creating positive training environments, we are going to have to use our voices and have some slightly uncomfortable conversations. In person feedback or even sending an email may feel pretty daunting. So, I've drafted a little template you can use:

'Dear _____,

Thank you for the workout today. I'm really enjoying working on getting fitter and stronger and I really appreciate your help.

However, it makes me feel uncomfortable when there is discussion of earning or burning food, and negative language is used to shame certain body types. I personally find it really motivating and uplifting when we talk about improving fitness, posture, strength, confidence and wellbeing. It would be really positive if there was a shift in the language used, as I would feel a lot happier coming back. I hope this feedback will be taken on board.

Thank you for listening.'

FINDING A PERSONAL TRAINER

I want to caveat this part by saying that having a personal trainer is not essential. However, if it suits your personality to have one-to-one guidance and you are fortunate enough to have the financial means to, I highly recommend working with someone who can help you train in a safe and effective way. Louise Green, author of the book *Big Fit Girl*, believes that we are the CEO of our own bodies, which I just love! She promotes advocating for yourself, especially when recruiting trainers and joining gyms or fitness studios. In her book, she talks about how, when we are looking to work with someone to help us with our physical and mental health, we should meet and treat the prospective expert as if it were a job interview. By taking charge and asking the right questions, we can make sure that we are working with someone who can offer the right kind of support. A good personal trainer will listen to and respect your questions and requests. Below, I've put together some key questions to consider asking when looking for a weight-inclusive PT. Alarm bells should be ringing if responses indicate that the trainer is resistant to focusing on performance based goals and insists that body composition should be the primary focus.

> » I don't want to be weighed or measured, as I would like to focus on getting fitter and stronger. How else would you track my progress?
> » What type of training do you specialize in? (strength, endurance, boxing, etc.)
> » Are you able to put me in touch with a qualified nutritionist or dietitian to assist with my nutrition if needed?
> » Do you believe that fit bodies come in all shapes and sizes?
> » How can you help me with my performance-based goals?

BODY DIVERSITY IN FITNESS

Or rather a severe lack of this, is a big problem. As a general population, we need to see more to be more. We need to see bodies of all shapes and sizes being included in media and marketing so that every body can feel included in fitness spaces. Not only is this a psychological barrier for people in larger bodies to overcome, for some there is a literal physical barrier of not being able to get through the turnstile at a local gym. We know how great the benefits of regular movement are for our mental and physical wellbeing, so why does the industry alienate so many people by marketing a narrow ideal of what fitness looks like?

When you steer away from traditional fitness model-type imagery and show a whole range of women moving in a whole variety of ways, it can be very powerful. The 'This Girl Can' campaign, which launched in 2015, has inspired almost three million women to get active. In their own words, 'This Girl Can celebrates active women who are doing their thing no matter how they do it, how they look or even how sweaty they get'. The campaign features imagery of women of all sizes, abilities, ages and ethnicities in motion, mid-workout, moving in a way that feels good! It's positive, it's powerful, it's not body shaming and it works. I hope the rest of the fitness industry catches on to the fact that when people feel included and welcome they are more likely to get involved. The mission of using drawings of bodies in this book, as well as a variety of models in the workout guide, is to remind us that fitness doesn't have a look or a size, everyone and every *body* is welcome.

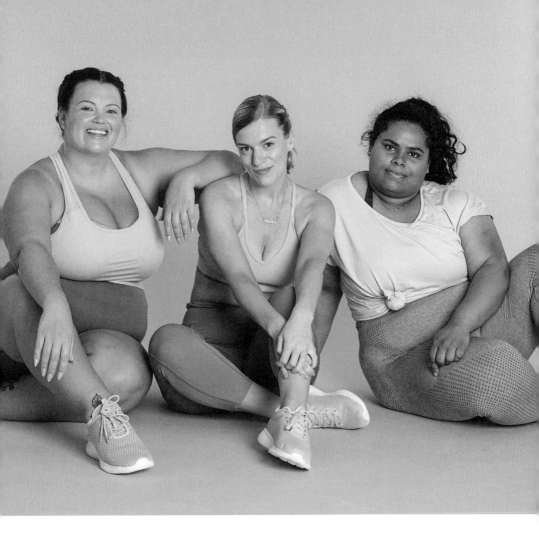

The lack of visible body diversity doesn't only hold people back from joining gyms, running groups or attending classes, it also makes budding personal trainers and instructors think twice about being a part of the industry. I have sadly had many interactions with people afraid to teach classes and train clients because they fear the judgements made upon their bodies. If that's you, if you're older or in a bigger body or don't feel you fit the fitness mould, let me say right now that we NEED you. We need fit people in all bodies, so that they can inspire other people who feel like outsiders to get involved too. We all have unique life experiences and perspectives, and the industry is better off with more of these in it.

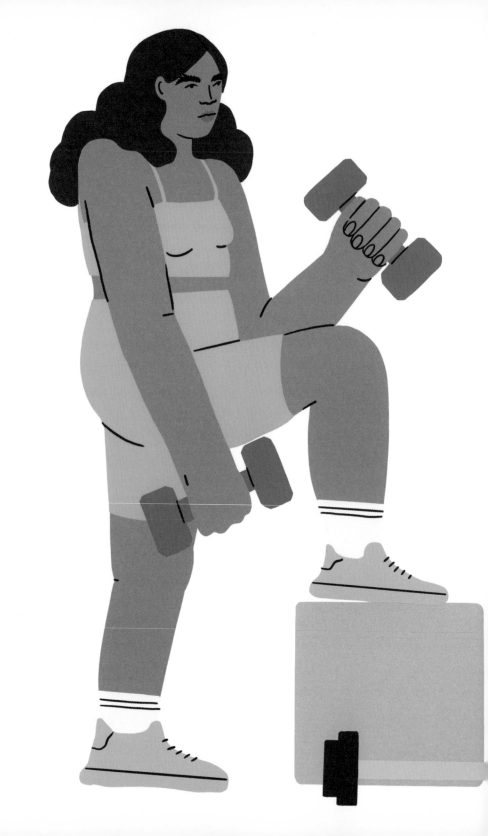

10 WEEKS TO TRAIN HAPPY

THE HAPPY + HEALTHY 10-WEEK WORKOUT PLAN

If you are new to the world of exercise, I hope that reading this book has taught you how wonderful movement is for the body and brain and inspired you to get started. If fitness is already a part of your life, I hope that this book has encouraged you to assess your relationship with it – is it making you feel happy and healthy?

ARE YOU READY?

Before embarking on this exercise plan, I would like you to consider the following questions that should help you decide if you are in the right headspace to begin a structured workout plan:

» Are my motivations to do this my own (intrinsic) as they should be, or are they still coming from external pressures (extrinsic)?
» Will I enjoy working out within this type of structure?
» Will I be kind to myself and allow myself flexibility if I use this guide?
» Am I ready for gentle guidance or are there a few more things I need to work through first?

Your answers will tell you if you're ready to start. There is no need to rush, in fact it is essential that you get to this stage of the book at your own pace and begin when you feel that the timing is right in the context of your life. You can also feel free to dip in and out or just stick to the parts that suit you best.

Whether you are a total beginner who needs a bit of guidance or a seasoned gym goer looking to bring back the fun and enjoy reconnecting with your body, I have designed this plan to be suitable for everyone. Tuning into your body to cultivate intuition with it is not an overnight process and it takes work, reflection and practice – 10 weeks is a good timeframe in which to do this. This is a resource that I hope will be useful for years to come, and you can repeat the steps or use it to build on the foundation you've created. My aim is to provide a gentle structure, allowing you space and time to explore and have fun finding different ways to move your body. So, let's get started!

HOW IT WORKS

Each week I've given you three types of workouts to complete. This simple structure allows room for you to have plenty of rest – and I must stress that it is imperative that you include a minimum of *1–2 rest days per week* or else you are probably in danger of overdoing it. From my experience, three times a week is a realistic amount for most people to aim for. If, for whatever reason, it feels like too much on certain weeks, then don't feel pressure to keep up and do them all. The most important thing is that you listen to your body and go at your own pace in order to practice intuitive exercise, having fun along the way. The three workouts are as follows:

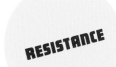

RESISTANCE TRAINING: The idea here is that you can invest in a few pieces of equipment and do the exercises in the comfort of your own home or outdoors, or make use of the equipment in your local gym. These full body workouts use kettlebells and dumbbells, and occasionally a bench or step. The difficulty level very gradually increases throughout the 10 weeks, and the aim is that by the end, you will be lifting heavier weights and completing more complex exercises as we build up your base strength.

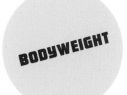

BODYWEIGHT TRAINING: These workouts don't require the use of any equipment, and so give you the freedom to train at home, outdoors or in the gym – no set up required. You will be doing a mixture of circuits, interval training and mobility workouts designed to build up strength, stamina and improve range of movement.

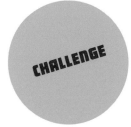

THE CHALLENGE: Each week, I've set you a challenge to find new and joyful ways of exercising and connecting to your body. These range from stretch and mobility sessions, to working out with a buddy and choosing a new form of movement to explore. At week 5 I have challenged you to set a personal best in an activity of your choice, and this is retested at week 10 as a way to monitor progress.

EQUIPMENT YOU WILL NEED:

- » Yoga mat
- » Dumbbells: light 2–4 kg/5–9 lb; medium 5–8 kg/10–17.5 lb; heavy 9 kg +/19 lb +
- » Kettlebells: light 4–6 kg/9–13 lb; medium 8–10 kg/17.5–22 lb; heavy 12 kg +/26 lb +
- » Bench or solid sturdy box
- » Chair or bench/box

Weights tip

With regards to your weight selection, choose weights that will challenge you on the last few reps of each exercise. You should be able to complete the exercises without drastically compromising form, but they should feel tough to do. I have indicated a ball-park range of what weight would suit best each exercise in the guide, but do use your own discretion and find what works best for you.

Timer tip

For a lot of these workouts an interval timer will be required. I use a free app called 'seconds' as it's really useful for inputting intervals.

Journal tip

I encourage you to use a notebook, workout log book or journal to track your progress with these workouts. You can then record the weights you have used for each exercise, as well as timings for finishers. You can also record your personal best information here and watch your progression over the 10 weeks. I would also like you to track how you *feel* in this journal – what was your mood before your workout and after? How has your self-esteem and body image improved each week? What does it feel like to get fitter and stronger?

You can find video demonstrations of each workout at:
www.tallyrye.co.uk/trainhappyvideos

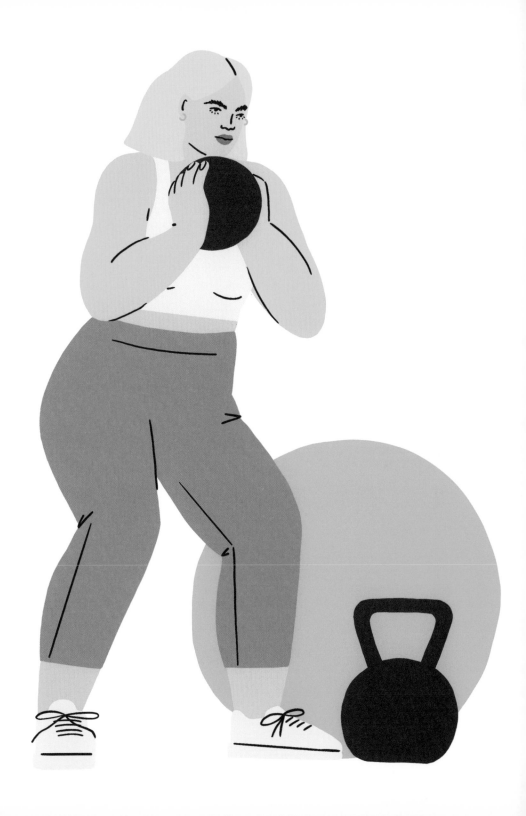

WARM-UP ROUTINE

The warm-up routine is just as important as the workout itself, as we are priming the body for movement. The aim of a warm-up is to activate your central nervous system with dynamic movements and raise your heart rate to get the warm blood flowing to your muscles. Warming up properly will reduce your risk of injury and maximize the range of movement you can reach in certain exercises, such as squats, which in turn makes your training more effective. Depending on your own body and its needs, you may like to spend more time on certain areas, but here is a simple and effective general warm-up routine to complete before each workout:

WALK OUT TO PLANK X 3

1.

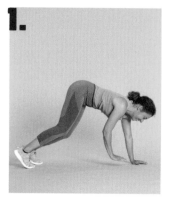
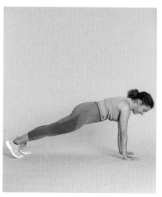

2.

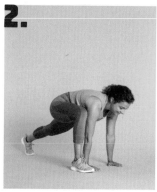
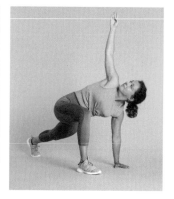

FULL MOUNTAIN CLIMBERS WITH T-SPINE ROTATION X 5 EACH SIDE

ALTERNATING LATERAL LUNGES WITH INSIDE FOOT TOUCHES X 10 EACH LEG

3.

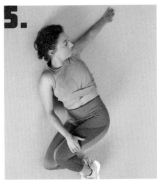

4.

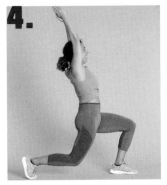

REVERSE LUNGES WITH OVERHEAD REACH X 5 EACH LEG

LYING LUMBAR SPINE TWISTS X 5 EACH SIDE

5.

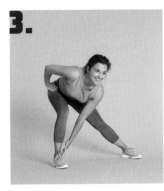

6.

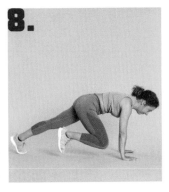

REVERSE PLANKS X 5

GLUTE BRIDGES 2 X SETS OF 15

7.

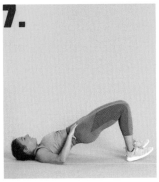

8.

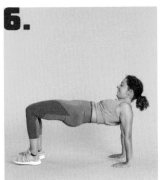

MOUNTAIN CLIMBERS 2 X SETS OF 20

STAR JUMPS 2 X SETS OF 10

9.

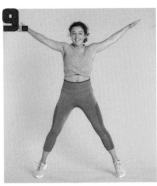

COOL-DOWN ROUTINE

A cool-down should be completed after every workout. The prime time for static stretches is post-training; these aim to lengthen the muscles, increase flexibility and aid in reducing DOMS (delayed onset muscle soreness). It's important to think about your breath and its connection to each stretch, using the exhale to sink deeper and relax into each position. Hold each stretch for 3 breaths in total. Breathe in for 4 (counting 1,2,3,4), take a slight pause, then exhale for 4 counts (4,3,2,1). If you have been doing more of a cardio-based session, you may like to include a gentle walk or cycle for 3–5 minutes to bring the heart rate down before moving into the stretches.

CHILD'S POSE
Right hand over left, then left hand over right

KNEELING ARM THREAD-THROUGHS
Right side, then left side

RIGHT LEG 90 DEGREES, BACK LEG EXTENDED
With hands inside leg, then elbows down

RIGHT PIGEON
Hands down, then elbows down with arms extended

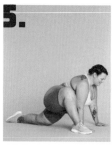
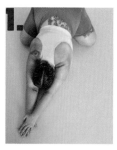
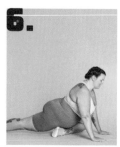
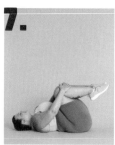
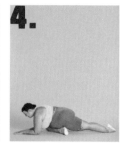
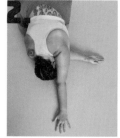
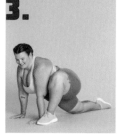
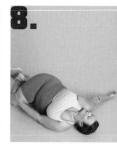

LEFT LEG 90 DEGREES, BACK LEG EXTENDED
With hands inside leg, then elbows down

LEFT PIGEON
Hands down, then elbows down with arms extended

LIE ON FLOOR
Hug knees in and rock from side to side

LIE ON FLOOR
Start with arms in T position; extend left leg, then hold right knee across body with left hand

LIE ON FLOOR

9.

Start with arms in T position; extend right leg, then hold left knee across body with right hand

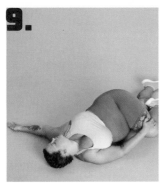

10.

UPWARD DOG

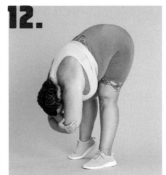

DOWNWARD DOG

11.

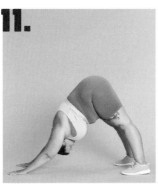

12.

RAG DOLL

Pop right knee, then pop left knee

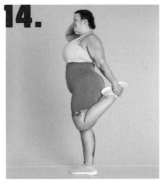

STANDING CHEST STRETCH

13.

Hands linked behind back

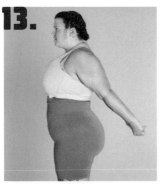

14.

STANDING QUAD STRETCH

Left leg, then right leg

15.

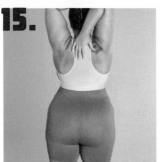

STANDING TRICEP STRETCH

Left arm, then right arm

WEEK 1

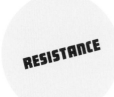

RESISTANCE

This week's workout is structured into supersets. A superset is when you complete two exercises back–to–back (for example, 8–10 goblet box squats followed straight away by 12 deadbugs). We start each workout with a compound move (one that works multiple muscle groups), this week it is the goblet box squat. The first exercise in each superset is the primary move and incorporates weights and the second exercise usually relies on bodyweight, though with the lunges you have the option to use one medium dumbbell. **The aim here is to complete two or three rounds of each superset, taking a 60–90 second rest between each round.**

1A.

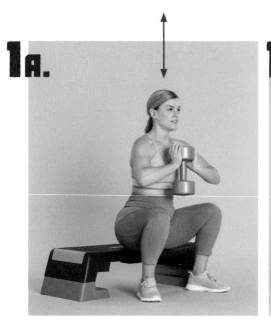

GOBLET BOX SQUAT
X 8-10

1 X HEAVY DUMBBELL
+ BENCH

1B.

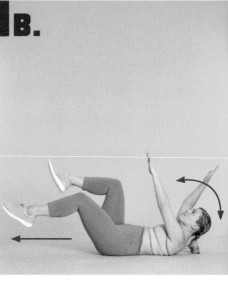

DEADBUGS
X 12

X3 SETS

2A.

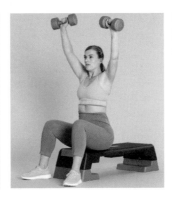

DUMBBELL SHOULDER PRESSES X 8-10

2 X MEDIUM DUMBBELLS

2B.

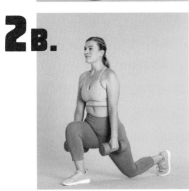

GOBLET REVERSE LUNGES X 8 EACH LEG

2 X MEDIUM DUMBBELLS

X2-3 SETS

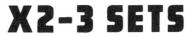

3A.

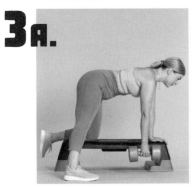

SINGLE ARM ROW X 8-10 EACH ARM

1 X MEDIUM DUMBBELL

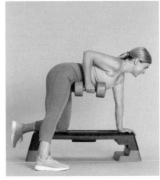

3B.

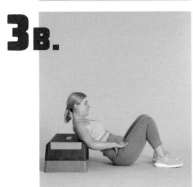

BODYWEIGHT HIP THRUSTS X 12-15

BENCH

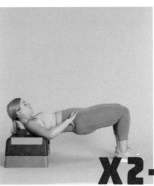

X2-3 SETS

4a.

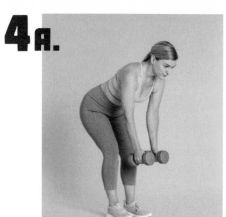
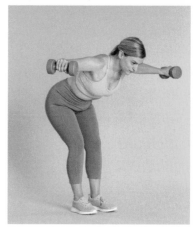

REVERSE FLYES X 10-12

2 X LIGHT DUMBBELLS

4b.

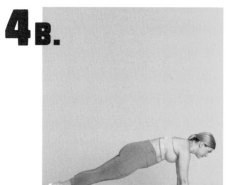
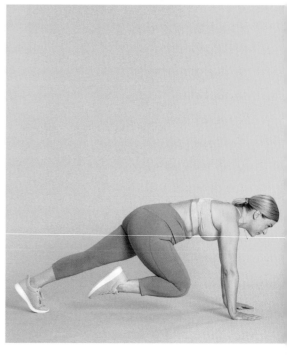

SLOW MOUNTAIN CLIMBERS X 20

X2 SETS

BODYWEIGHT

This is a circuit made up of 6 exercises. **Work for 30 seconds per exercise, then rest for 30 seconds. Complete three–four rounds of the circuit, taking 60–90 seconds of rest at the end of each.**

1.

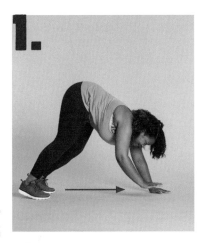 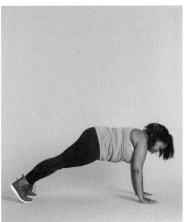

WALK OUT TO PLANK

2.

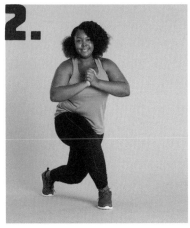 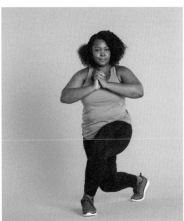

CURTSEY LUNGES

3-4 ROUNDS

3.

BACK RAISES

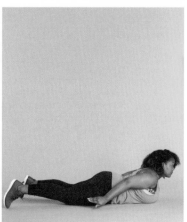
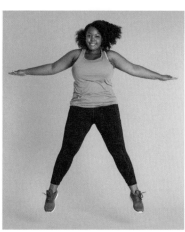

4.

ICE SKATERS

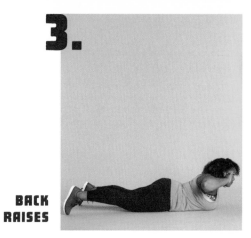
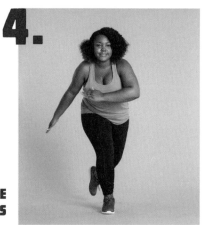
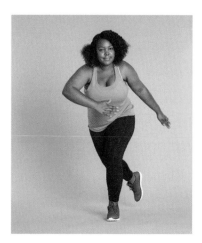

5.

**GLUTE
BRIDGES**

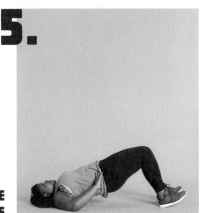

6.

**PLANK TO
SQUATS**

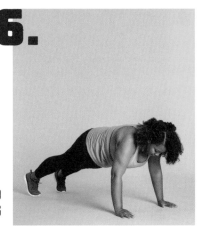

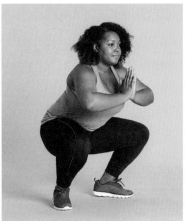

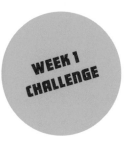

**WEEK 1
CHALLENGE**

Everyday Active! Try and sneak an extra 20 minutes more movement into your every day. That might be taking the stairs, going for a walk on your lunch break or parking further away from where you need to be. Think about how you can incorporate movement in a way that makes you feel good, and gives you a bit of headspace this week.

WEEK 2

This workout is again structured into superset pairs. This week the focus is on the sumo deadlift as our compound move. As with week 1, complete the two exercises in each superset back to back. **Complete three rounds of each superset, taking a 60–90 second rest between each round.**

RESISTANCE

1A.

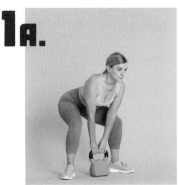
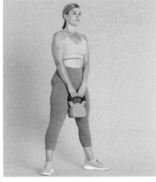

SUMO DEADLIFTS X 10

1 X HEAVY KETTLEBELL

1B.

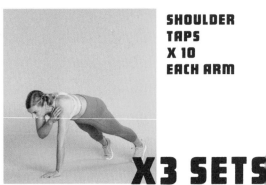

SHOULDER TAPS X 10 EACH ARM

X3 SETS

2A.

GOBLET CURTSEY LUNGES X 8 EACH LEG
1 X MEDIUM DUMBBELL

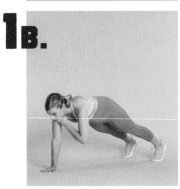

2B.

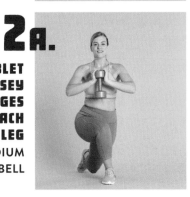
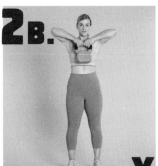

UPRIGHT ROWS X 10-12

1 X MEDIUM KETTLEBELL

X3 SETS

3A.

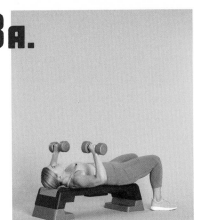 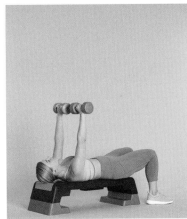

CHEST PRESSES

2 X MEDIUM
DUMBBELLS +
BENCH

3B.

DEADBUGS

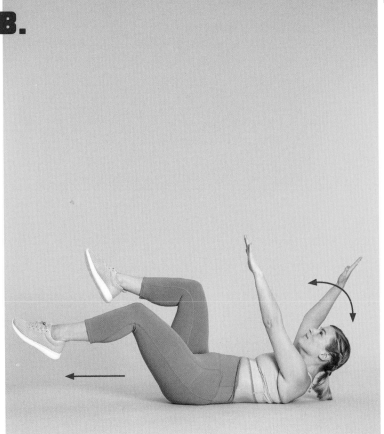

X3 SETS

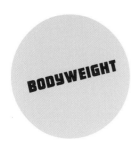

BODYWEIGHT

This is a workout of two halves: lower body and upper body. There are two circuits with four exercises each. **Work for 30 seconds per exercise, then rest for 15 seconds. Complete three rounds of each circuit, taking 60–90 seconds of rest at the end of each.**

LOWER BODY CIRCUIT

SPLIT LUNGES (RIGHT LEG)

SPLIT LUNGES (LEFT LEG)

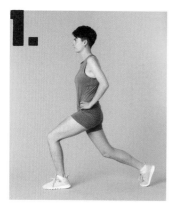

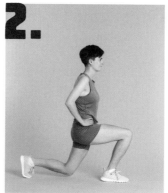

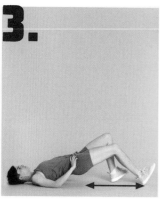

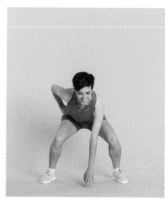

HAMSTRING WALKOUTS

CRISS–CROSS SQUAT JUMPS

3 ROUNDS

ECCENTRIC PRESS-UPS *KNEELING

TRICEP DIPS

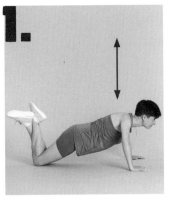

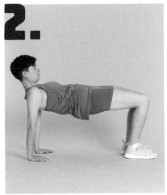

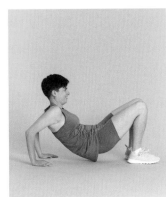

3.

4.

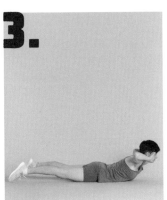

BACK RAISES

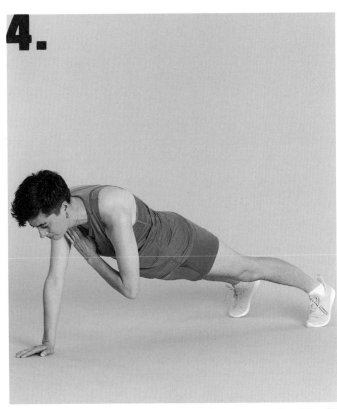

PLANK SHOULDER TAPS + KNEE TAPS

3 ROUNDS

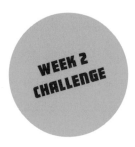

WEEK 2 CHALLENGE

Get Mobile! It's important to think about our mobility. The more mobile our joints and flexible our muscles, the more we can get out of exercises. It will help things like your squats get deeper, your lunges lower and your shoulders less restricted. Aim to do this mobility routine at least once this week and feel the difference. You might like to film or take pictures of yourself doing the routine as a way to track your how your posture and mobility progress.

YOGA FLOW X 5

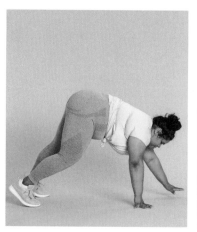

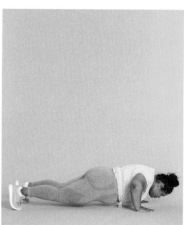

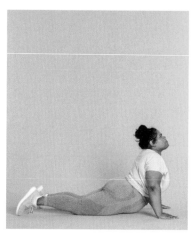

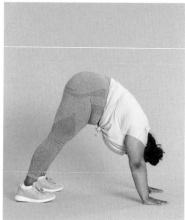

FULL MOUNTAIN CLIMBERS WITH T-SPINE ROTATION X 10 EACH SIDE

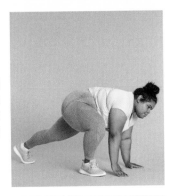 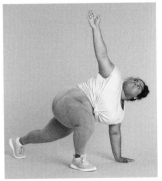

SCAPULA WALL SLIDES X 10

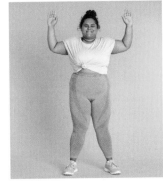 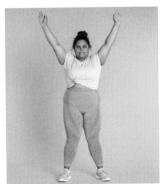

KNEELING PLANK WITH SINGLE ARM 'SWIMMERS' X 10 EACH ARM

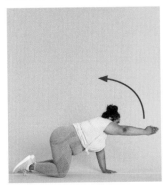 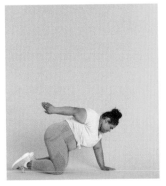

WIDE CHILD'S POSE + SINGLE LEG CHILD'S POSE X 5 EACH LEG

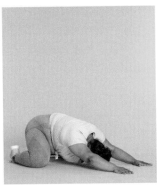 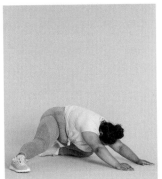

WEEK 3

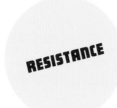

RESISTANCE

This week, the workout is comprised of two tri-sets rounded off with a finisher. The first tri-set (1A, 1B, 1C) focuses on completing three consecutive push-based exercises, whilst the second tri–set (2A, 2B, 2C) is made up of three consecutive pull-based exercises. We end with a pyramid finisher, which is comprised of two exercises. Each exercise starts with a high number of reps, which gradually decreases for each set. **Complete three lots of the push tri-set, with 60–90 seconds between each set, before moving on to three rounds of the pull tri-set. Complete the pyramid finisher as quickly (and safely) as possible with minimal rest.**

1A.

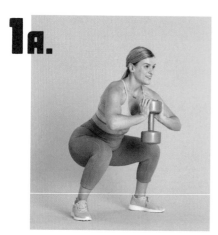

GOBLET SQUATS X 8-10

1 X HEAVY DUMBBELL

1B.

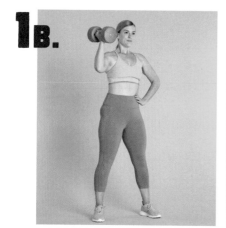 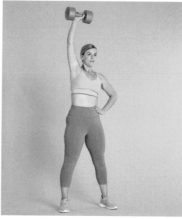

SINGLE ARM SHOULDER PRESSES X 8-10 EACH ARM

1 X MEDIUM DUMBBELL

1c.

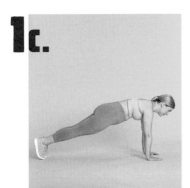
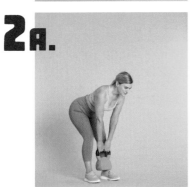

SLOW MOUNTAIN CLIMBERS X 20

X3 SETS

2A.

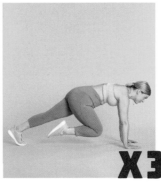

ROMANIAN DEADLIFTS X 8-10

1 X HEAVY KETTLEBELL

2B.

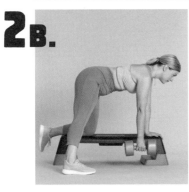
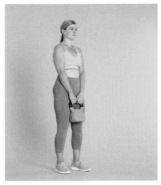

SINGLE ARM ROWS X 8-10 EACH ARM

1 X MEDIUM DUMBBELL

2C.

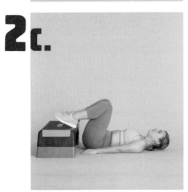
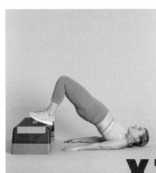

BODYWEIGHT HIP THRUSTS X 15

BENCH

X3 SETS

FINISHER

A.

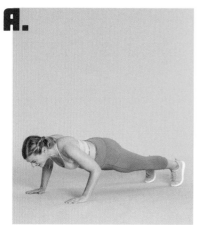 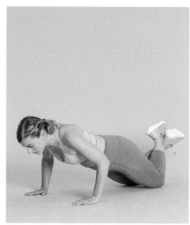

**PRESS-UPS
X 12/8/4**

B.

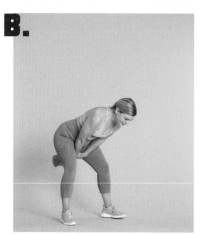 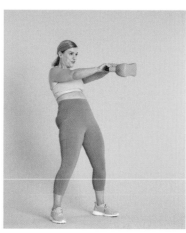

**KETTLEBELL
SWINGS
X 15/10/5**

1 X MEDIUM
KETTLEBELL

X3 SETS

This time, the bodyweight workout is divided into supersets (two consecutive exercises), with the theme being strength + sweat! The first exercise in each pair is resistance-based, whilst the second exercise raises your heart rate. **Work for 40 seconds, then rest for 20 seconds and complete each superset four times before moving on to the next set.** Of course, if four rounds is too much, then switch to three rounds for this week.

1A.

SUMO SQUATS

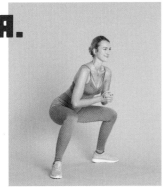

1B.

WALKOUTS TO FULL MOUNTAIN CLIMBER

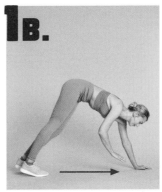

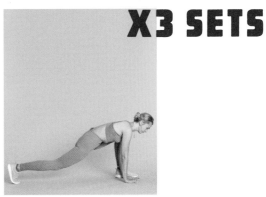

X3 SETS

2A.

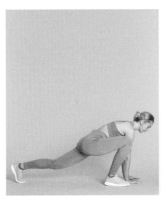

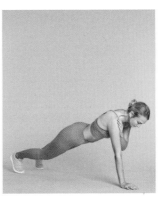

SHOULDER TAPS

2B.

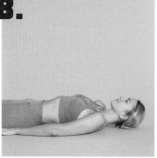

LIE DOWN, STAND UP

X3 SETS

3A.

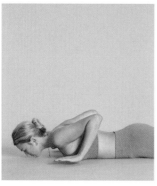

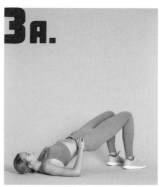

T-GLUTE BRIDGES

3B.

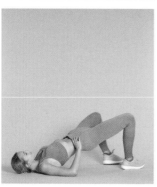

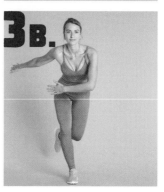

ICE SKATERS

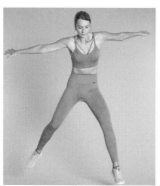

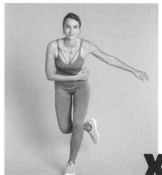

X3 SETS

4A.

DEADBUGS

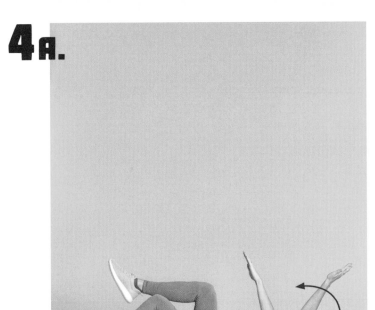

4B.

LATERAL HIGH KNEES

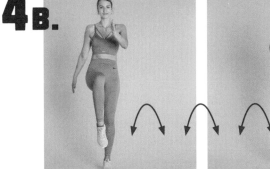
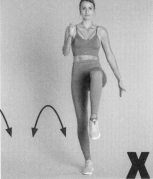

X3 SETS

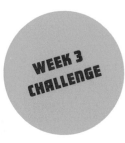

WEEK 3 CHALLENGE

Try something new... This week, I want you to find a NEW and exciting way to move your body – something you've never done before! Perhaps you might like to do a new class? Join a running club? Check out your local sports teams? The exercise world is your oyster.

WEEK 4

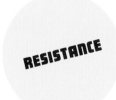
This week's resistance workout follows a similar structure to week 3. Once again, we have two tri–sets, followed by a finisher. The primary exercise in the first tri–set is the sumo deadlift, so this is the one to go heaviest on. **Complete three rounds of each tri–set, with 60–90 seconds between each round. The finisher for today's workout is a one song AMRAP – choose your favourite workout song, and aim to complete as many rounds as possible of the three exercises listed.** Be sure to note how many you do down for future reference.

1A.

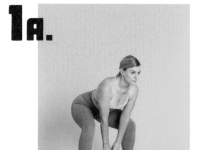
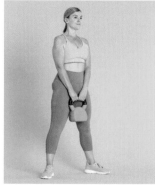

SUMO DEADLIFTS X 8-10

1 X HEAVY KETTLEBELL

1B.

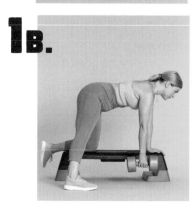
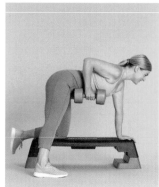

SINGLE ARM ROWS X 20–24 (10–12 EACH ARM)

MEDIUM DUMBBELL

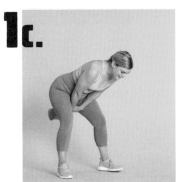

1c.

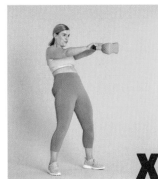

KETTLEBELL SWINGS X 15

MEDIUM
KETTLEBELL

X3 SETS

2A.

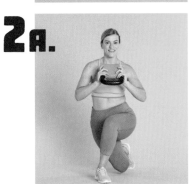

GOBLET CURTSEY LUNGES X 16-20

1 X MEDIUM
KETTLEBELL

2B.

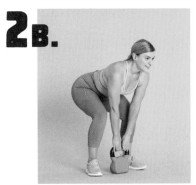

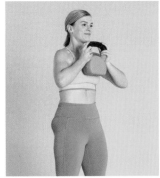

KETTLEBELL SQUATS, CLEAN + PRESS X 8-12

LIGHT OR
MEDIUM
KETTLEBELL

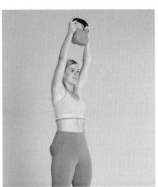

2c.

SLOW FULL MOUNTAIN CLIMBERS X 16-20

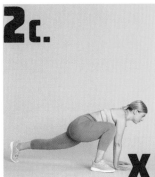

X3 SETS

FINISHER

A. 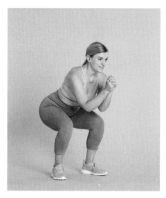 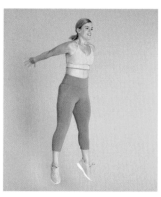 **SQUAT JUMPS X 8**

B. 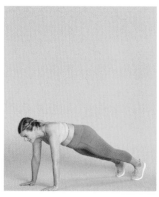 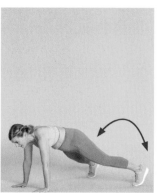 **PLANK JACKS X 16**

C. 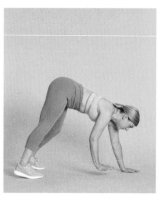 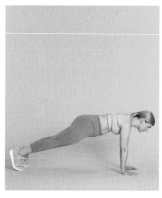 **WALK OUT TO PLANK X 10**

AS MANY ROUNDS AS POSSIBLE FOR 1 SONG!

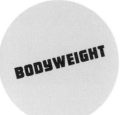

BODYWEIGHT

Here we have three exercise pyramids, each with a different focus: mobility, strength and cardio. **Complete four rounds of each tri–set, completing the exercises back-to-back with opportunity to rest for 60 seconds at the end of each round.**

MOBILITY

1a.

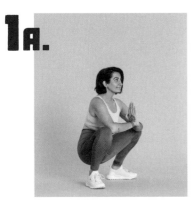
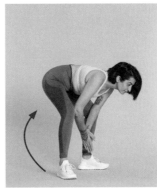

**FROG
SQUATS
X 5**

1b.

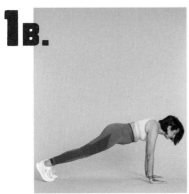
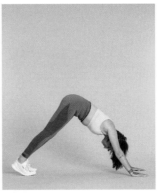

**PLANK TO
DOWNWARD
DOG
X 10**

1c.

X4 SETS

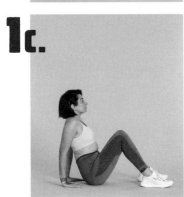
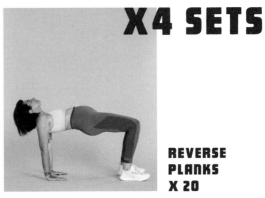

**REVERSE
PLANKS
X 20**

2A.

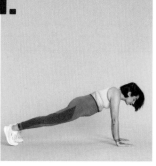 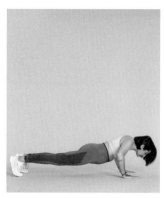

ECCENTRIC PRESS-UPS X 5

2B.

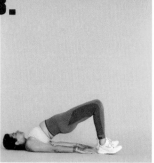 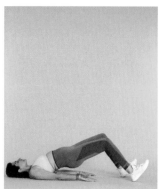

HAMSTRING WALKOUTS X 10

2C.

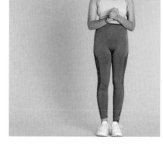 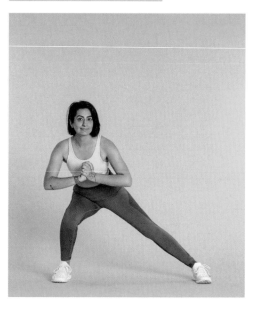

LATERAL LUNGES X 20

X4 SETS

CARDIO

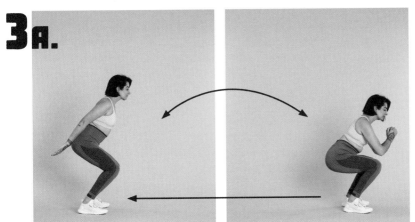

3A.

FORWARD BOUNDS + RUN BACK X 12

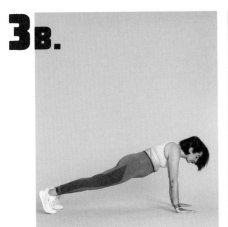

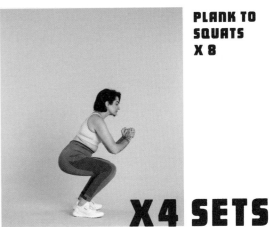

3B.

PLANK TO SQUATS X 8

X4 SETS

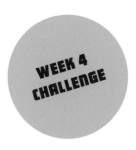

WEEK 4 CHALLENGE

Get outdoors and explore! There are so many benefits to getting active in nature. I challenge you to walk or run to a local (or distant) beauty spot or area of interest and soak it all in. As always, I encourage you to get friends and family involved if you can. Going for a walk in the park or a hike up a mountain is a fab way to hang out with friends whilst enjoying nature and staying active.

WEEK 5

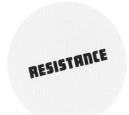
This week, we are upping the intensity of the resistance workout by following a new structure; a superset, followed by two tri–sets. As we are at week 5, I encourage you to start increasing the weights used where you can, for example, if you can comfortably do 10 reps of a goblet squat, try slightly increasing the weight and aiming for eight reps to start with. **Complete three sets of the superset and two tri–sets, taking 60–90 seconds between each round.** The last few reps of each exercise should feel challenging to complete.

1A.

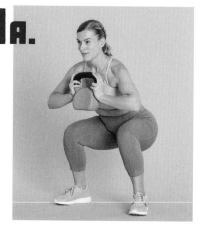

PAUSE GOBLET SQUATS X 8-10

1 X HEAVY KETTLEBELL

1B.

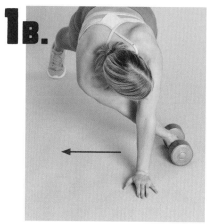
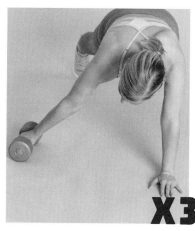

PLANK DUMBBELL PULL-THROUGHS X 16-20

1 X MEDIUM DUMBBELL

X3 SETS

2A.

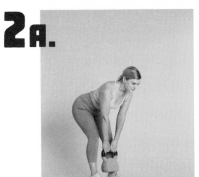
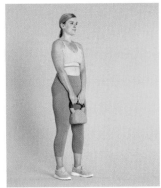

ROMANIAN DEADLIFTS X 8-10

1 X HEAVY KETTLEBELL

2B.

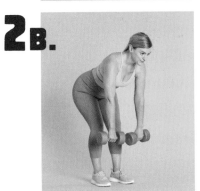
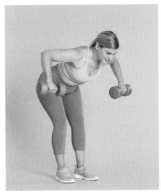

BENT OVER WIDE ROWS X 10-12

2 X LIGHT OR MEDIUM DUMBBELLS

2C.

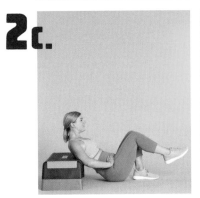
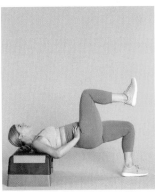

SINGLE LEG HIP THRUSTS X 10 EACH LEG

BENCH

X2 SETS

3A.

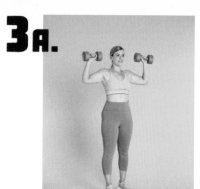
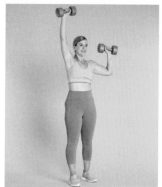

ALTERNATING STANDING DUMBBELL PRESSES X 6 EACH ARM

2 X MEDIUM DUMBBELLS

3B.

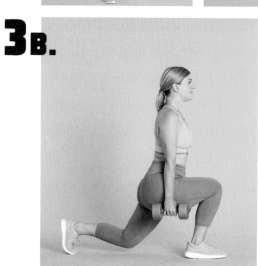

ALTERNATING WALKING LUNGES (LONG STRIDE) X 20

2 X MEDIUM DUMBBELLS

3C.

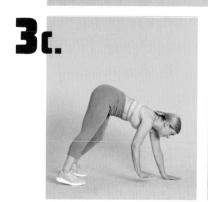
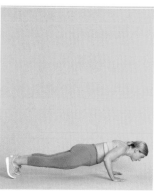

WALKOUT TO PRESS-UPS X 10

X2 SETS

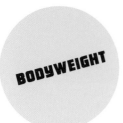

BODYWEIGHT

We are back to our bodyweight circuit, and this week we have increased the number of exercises to eight and the work time. **Work for 40 seconds on each exercise, then rest for 20 seconds, taking 30–90 seconds rest between three–four rounds of each circuit.**

FORWARD BOUND + RUN BACKS

1.

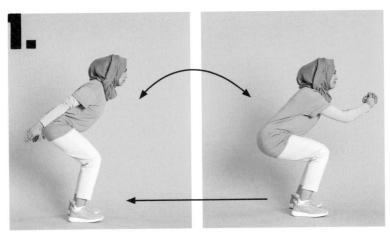

2.

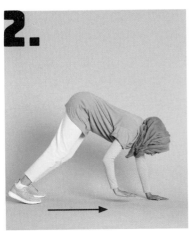
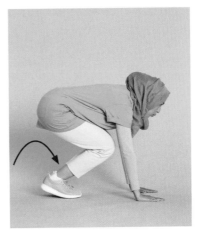

WALK OUT TO THRUSTERS

X 3-4 SETS

3.

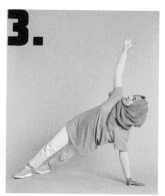

**PLANK
T-TWISTS**

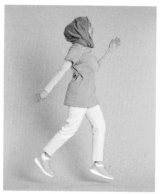

4.

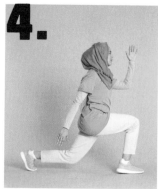

**1 + 1/2
JUMPING
LUNGES**

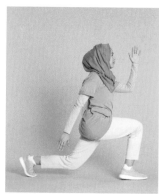

5.

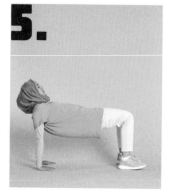

**TRICEP
DIPS**

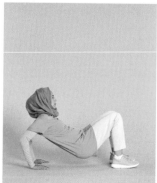

CURTSEY LUNGES

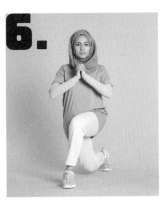

LATERAL BEAR CRAWLS

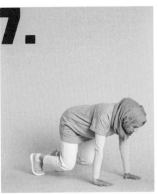
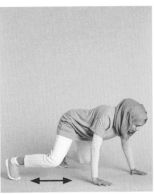

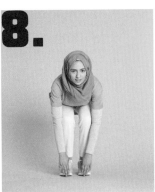

EXPLOSIVE STAR JUMPS

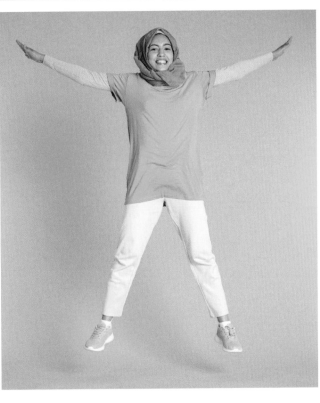

Set a new personal best! Choose an activity you enjoy and try to set a new personal best. It can be anything from the longest distance you've ever run, to the fastest you've ever swum lengths, the heaviest weight you've ever lifted or how many press-ups you can do. It is best to go with something you enjoy, as we will return to this later on in the guide to check your progress.

WEEK 5 CHALLENGE

WEEK 6

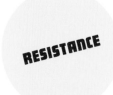

RESISTANCE

The structure of the week six workout is the same as week five. The heaviest exercise for this session will be the parallel deadlift, as we are using two heavy kettlebells. **Aim to complete three rounds of the superset and the two tri-sets, taking 60–90 seconds of rest between each round.**

1A.

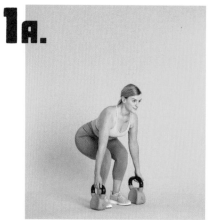

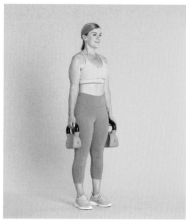

PARALLEL DEADLIFTS X 8-10

2 X HEAVY KETTLEBELLS

1B.

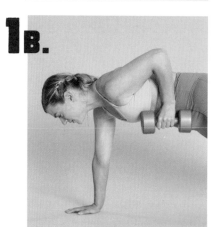

PLANK ROWS X 20

1 X MEDIUM DUMBBELL

X3 SETS

2a.

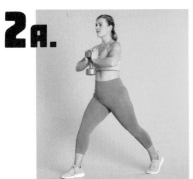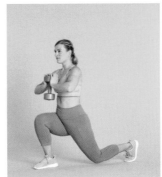

SPLIT GOBLET LUNGES X 10 EACH LEG

1 X MEDIUM DUMBBELL

2b.

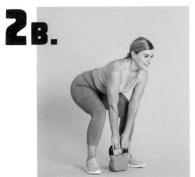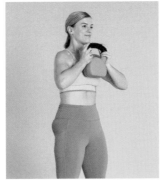

SQUAT, CLEAN + PRESS X 10-12

1 X MEDIUM KETTLEBELL

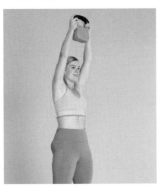

2c.

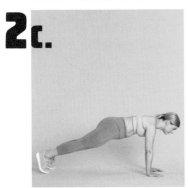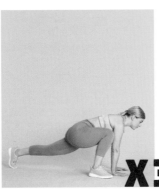

X CLIMBERS X 20

X3 SETS

3A.

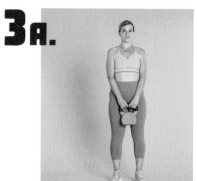
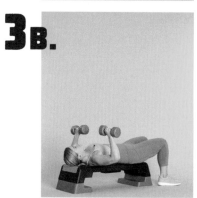

LATERAL LUNGES X 20

1 X MEDIUM KETTLEBELL

3B.

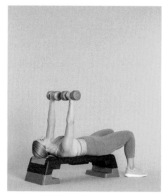
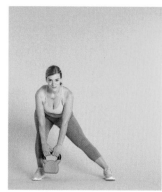

CHEST PRESSES X 10-12

2 X MEDIUM DUMBBELLS + BENCH

3C.

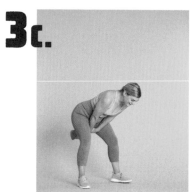
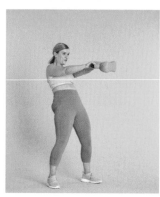

KETTLEBELL SWINGS X 15-20

1 X MEDIUM KETTLEBELL

X3 SETS

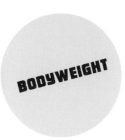

We are back to doing the upper and the lower body circuits, but this time incorporating a chair (or box/bench if at the gym). Start with the lower body circuit and then move on to the upper body. **For each circuit, work for 40 seconds on and 20 seconds off, and complete three or four rounds, taking 60–90 seconds of rest between each round.**

LOWER BODY CIRCUIT

BULGARIAN SPLIT LUNGES (LEFT LEG)

BULGARIAN SPLIT LUNGES (RIGHT LEG)

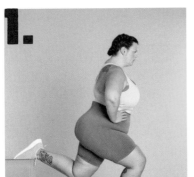

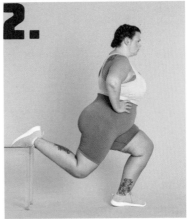

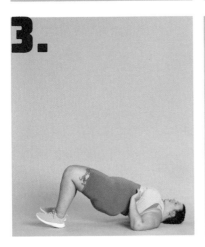

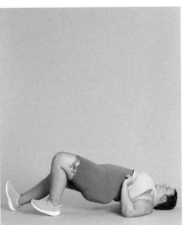

HAMSTRING WALKOUTS

4.

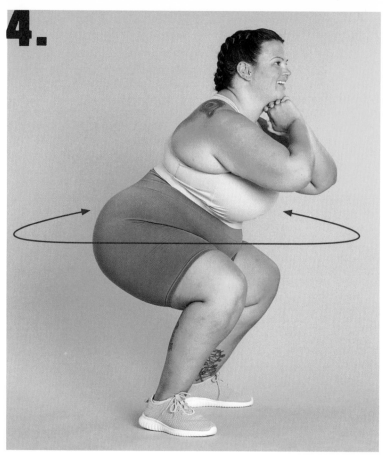

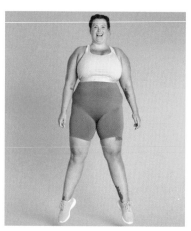

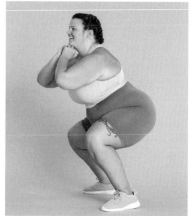

**180- DEGREE
SQUAT JUMPS**

X3-4 SETS

TRAVELLING PRESS-UPS (KNEELING)

LYING BACK RAISES

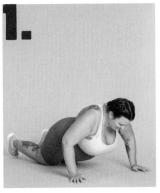

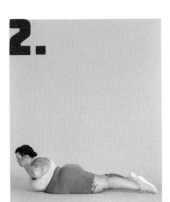

1.

2.

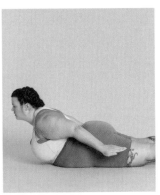

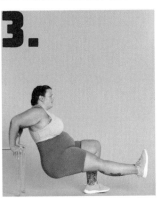

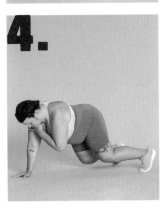

3.

4.

SINGLE LEG TRICEP DIPS WITH CHAIR

BEAR PLANK + SHOULDER TAPS

X3-4 SETS

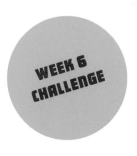

WEEK 6 CHALLENGE

Buddy up! This week, I challenge you to join forces with a friend to do your workout! To help make fitness fun, let's make it social too. Choose a workout of your choice such as a dance class, swimming, hiking, yoga, running (or whatever you like) and do it together. It's a great way to both stay active, and catch up.

WEEK 7

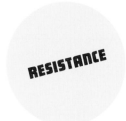

RESISTANCE

For this session there are two tri–sets followed by a pyramid finisher. We are used to this structure now, but I have programmed the exercises to be slightly more difficult than previous weeks. **Aim to do three rounds of each tri–set before completing the pyramid finisher. As before, complete the five rounds of pyramid exercises back-to-back with minimal rest.** If you want to track your progress with these, time yourself and note it down in your exercise journal.

1A.

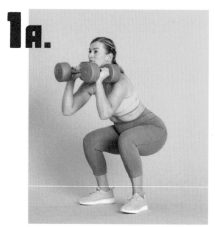

FRONT RACK SQUATS X 8-10

2 X MEDIUM DUMBBELLS

1B.

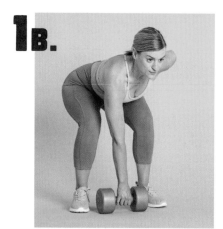

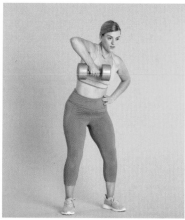

SINGLE ARM DUMBBELL SNATCHES X 8–10 EACH ARM

1 X MEDIUM DUMBBELL

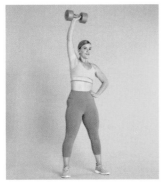
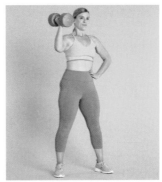

1c.

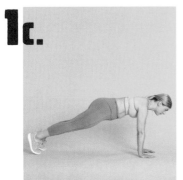
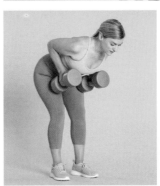

**PLANK
KNEE
TAPS
X 16-20**

X3 SETS

2a.

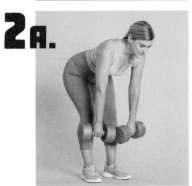
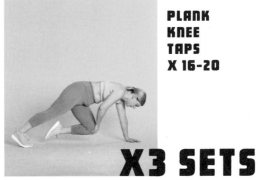

**ROMANIAN
DEADLIFTS
+ ROW
X 10-12**

2 X MEDIUM
DUMBBELLS

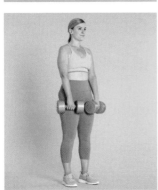

2B.

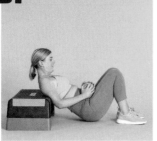

DUMBBELL HIP THRUSTS X 10-12

1 X MEDIUM OR HEAVY DUMBBELL

2C.

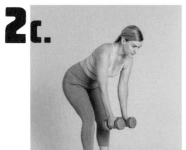
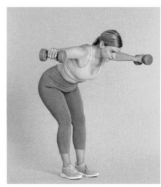

REVERSE FLYES X 12

2 X LIGHT DUMBBELLS

X3 SETS

FINISHER

A.

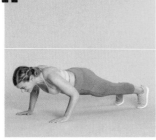
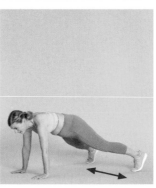

PRESS-UPS + PLANK JACKS X 10, 8, 6, 4, 2

B.

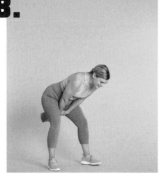
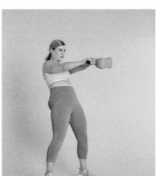

KETTLEBELL SWINGS X 20, 16, 12, 8, 4

1 X KETTLEBELL

X5 SETS

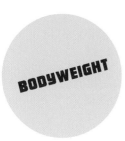

BODYWEIGHT

Back to the strength and sweat supersets for this week's workout but this time we are increasing the number of rounds completed. **Complete the two exercises in each superset for 40 seconds on, 20 seconds off, for eight rounds in total this time. Take 60–90 seconds of rest between each superset.**

1A.

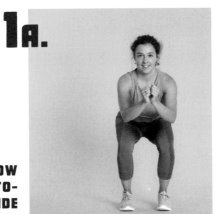
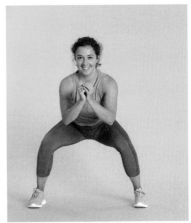

NARROW -TO- WIDE SQUATS

1B.

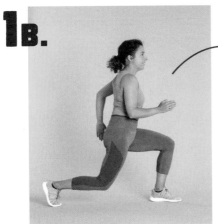
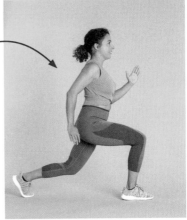

JUMPING LUNGES + PULSE

2A.

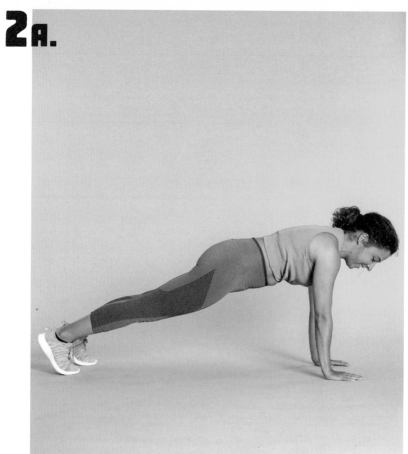

**PRESS-UPS
+ SHOULDER
TAPS**

2B.

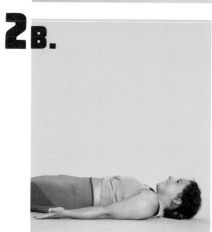 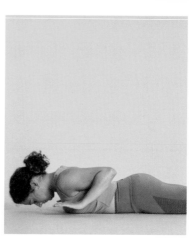

**LIE DOWN,
STAND UP**

3A.

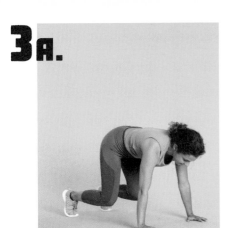 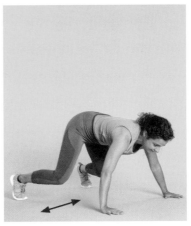

LATERAL BEAR CRAWLS

3B.

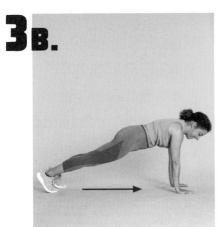 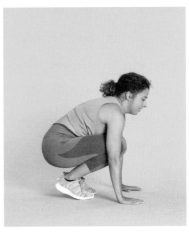

WALKOUTS TO PLANK THRUSTER

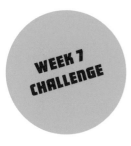

WEEK 7 CHALLENGE

Sign up for a challenge! Find a local event in your area that you can sign up to do in the future. Perhaps it's a charity 5K run or walk? An obstacle course? A special hike? Or a Zumbathon? There are lots of great things to choose from, and even better when you can use it as an opportunity to support a charity too. Doing good for you and for your community.

WEEK 8

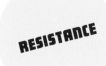

RESISTANCE

This week we up the ante to two giant sets, that are each made up of four exercises done consecutively. The first giant set is our 'pull' circuit and the second giant set is our 'push' circuit. **Aim to complete three–four rounds of each giant set, taking one–two minutes of rest between each complete round.**

1A.

SUMO DEADLIFTS X 8-10

1 X MEDIUM OR HEAVY KETTLEBELL

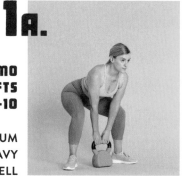

1B.

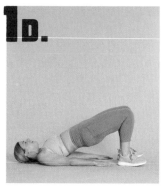

GOBLET CURTSEY LUNGES X 16-20

1 X MEDIUM OR HEAVY KETTLEBELL

1C.

BENT OVER ROWS X 10-12

2 X MEDIUM DUMBBELLS

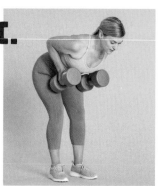

1D.

GLUTE BRIDGES X 12-15

X3-4 SETS

2A.

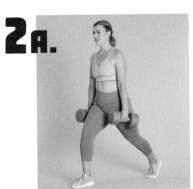
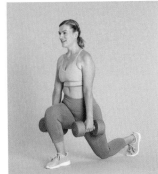

WALKING LUNGES X 10 EACH LEG

2 X MEDIUM OR HEAVY KETTLEBELLS

2B.

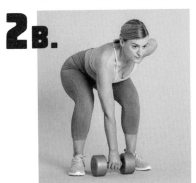
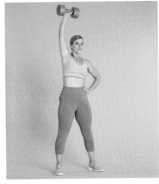

SINGLE ARM DUMBBELL SNATCHES X 10 EACH ARM

1 X MEDIUM DUMBBELL

2C.

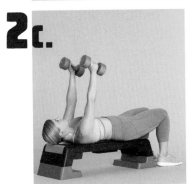
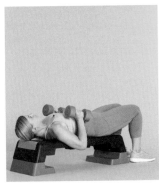

TRICEP CHEST PRESSES X 10-12

BENCH + 2 X LIGHT OR MEDIUM DUMBBELLS

2D.

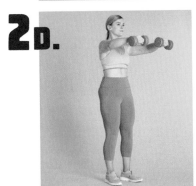
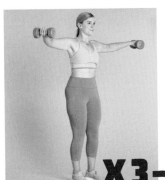

FRONT-TO-LATERAL RAISES X 10-12

2 X LIGHT DUMBBELLS

X3-4 SETS

BODYWEIGHT

For week 8, we are revisiting our mobility, strength and cardio pyramids. **The aim is to complete the three exercises within the pyramid back-to-back, taking 45–60 seconds rest between each round and completing five rounds of each pyramid in total.**

MOBILITY

1A.

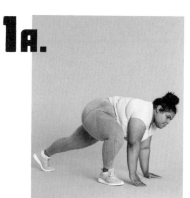
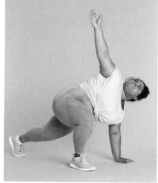

ALTERNATING FULL MOUNTAIN CLIMBERS + T-TWISTS X 20

1B.

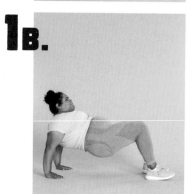

REVERSE PLANKS X 15

X5 SETS

1C.

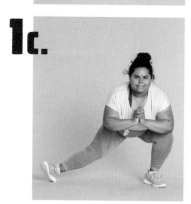
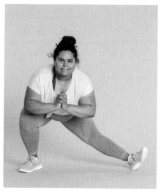

COSSACK SQUATS X 10

STRENGTH

2a.

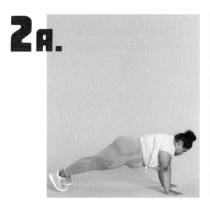
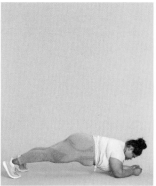

**COMMANDO
PLANKS
X 8**

2b.

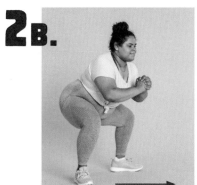
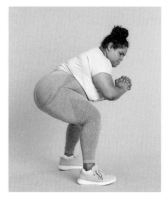

**SQUAT DUCK
WALKS
X 12**

2c.

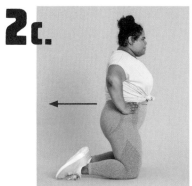
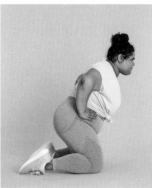

**KNEELING
GOOD
MORNINGS
X 15**

X5 SETS

CARDIO

3A.

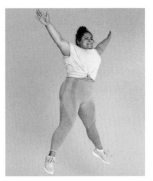

EXPLOSIVE STAR JUMPS X 5

3B.

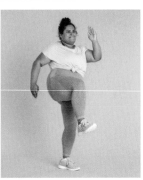

WALKOUT BURPEES X 10

3C.

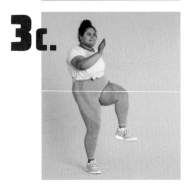

HIGH KNEES WITH A PAUSE X 30

X5 SETS

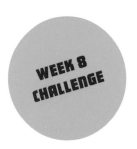

WEEK 8 CHALLENGE

Try something new…again! I encourage you to choose something that involves booking out the time in your diary to you make sure that you attend. If you need some ideas check out page 53 for inspiration.

WEEK 9

RESISTANCE

For the opening superset in this week's workout we are increasing the target as we work on upping the intensity in the final weeks. **Complete four rounds of each superset, then three rounds of each tri-set. As usual, take 60–90 seconds to rest between each round.**

1A.

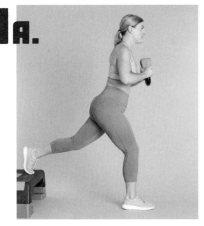

GOBLET BULGARIAN SPLIT LUNGES X 8 EACH LEG

BENCH +
1 X MEDIUM
KETTLEBELL

1B.

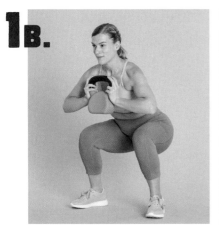

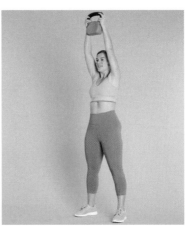

KETTLEBELL CLEANS + PRESSES X 8-10

1 X MEDIUM
KETTLEBELL

X4 SETS

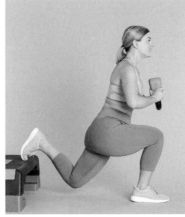

2A.

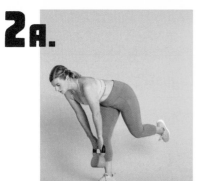
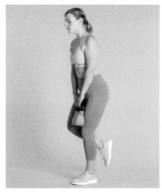

SINGLE LEG ROMANIAN DEAD LIFTS X 8–10 EACH LEG

1 X HEAVY OR MEDIUM KETTLEBELL

2B.

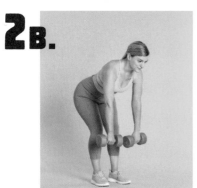
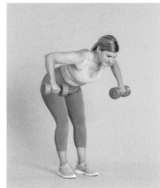

WIDE BENT OVER ROWS X 10-12

2 X MEDIUM DUMBBELLS

2C.

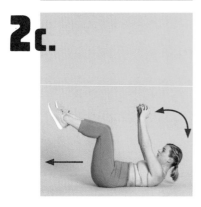
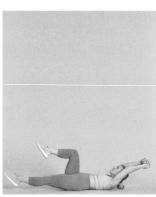

TWO-HAND DEADBUGS X 12

1 X LIGHT DUMBBELL

X3 SETS

3A.

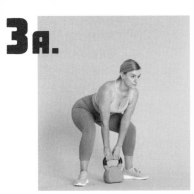
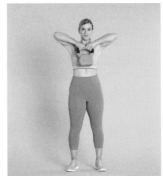

**SQUAT +
UPRIGHT
ROWS
X 12**

1 X MEDIUM
OR HEAVY
KETTLEBELL

3B.

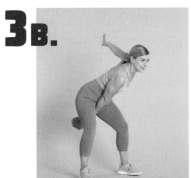
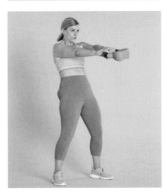
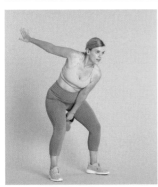

**SINGLE-ARM
KETTLEBELL
SWINGS
X 15**

1 X MEDIUM
KETTLEBELL

3C.

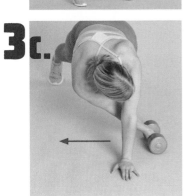
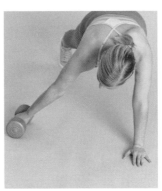

**PLANK
PULL-
THROUGHS
X 20**

1 X MEDIUM
DUMBBELL

X3 SETS

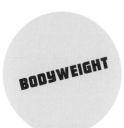

BODYWEIGHT

To increase the level of this week's bodyweight workout, we are aiming to do **five rounds of the eight exercises with 45 seconds on and 15 seconds off. Of course, please take 60–90 seconds of rest between each completed circuit.**

1.

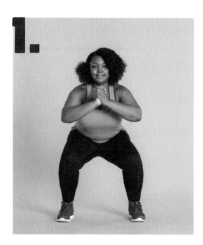

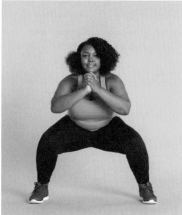

NARROW -TO- WIDE SQUAT JUMPS

2.

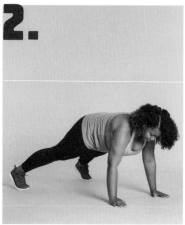

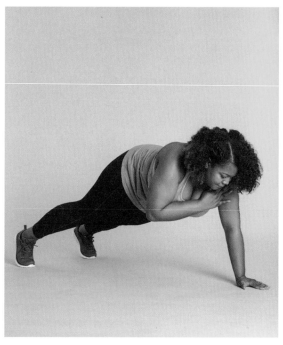

4 PLANK JACKS + 4 SHOULDER TAPS

3.

JACK KNIVES

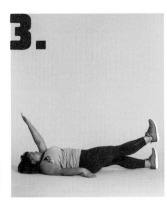
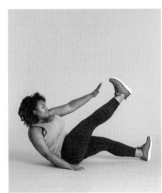

4.

REVERSE LUNGES TO SINGLE LEG HOPS

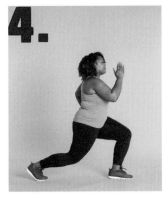
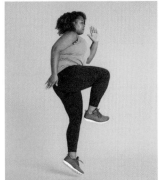

5.

BREAKDANCER PLANK

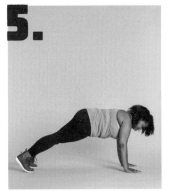
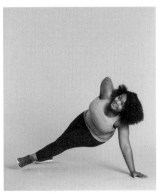

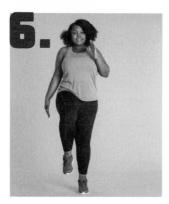
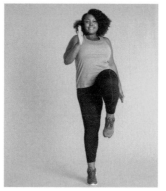

LATERAL HIGH KNEES

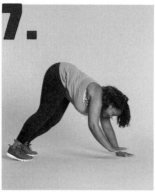
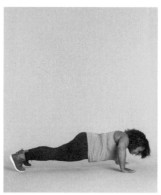

WALK OUT TO 3 PRESS-UPS

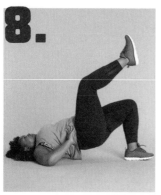
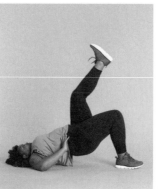

GLUTE BRIDGE KICKS

X5 SETS

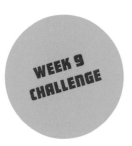

WEEK 9 CHALLENGE

Write your own workout! Write your own workout based on the exercises we have done for the past nine weeks and the structure we have used. Get creative, design a workout you will enjoy and have fun with it!

WEEK 10

Three tri–sets this week, with the first focusing on pull exercises, the second on push-based exercises. As you know by now, **complete each exercise within the tri–set back-to-back before resting for 60–90 seconds. Aim to do three rounds of each tri–set.**

1A.

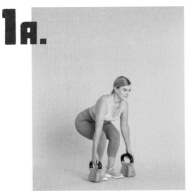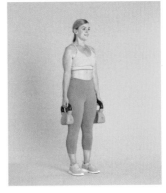

PARALLEL DEADLIFTS X 8-10

2 X HEAVY KETTLEBELLS

1B.

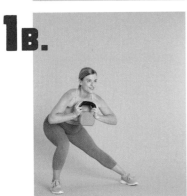

GOBLET LATERAL LUNGES X 8 EACH LEG

1 X MEDIUM KETTLEBELL

1c.

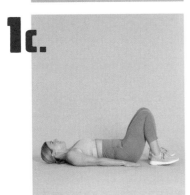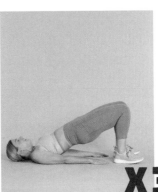

GLUTE BRIDGES X 15

X3 SETS

2A.

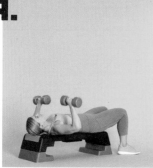
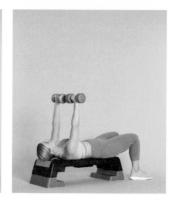

CHEST PRESSES X 10-12

BENCH +
2 X MEDIUM
DUMBBELLS

2B.

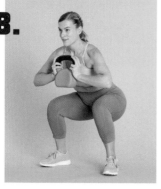
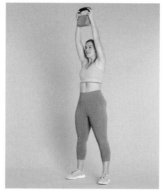

SQUATS + PRESS X 10-12

1 X MEDIUM
KETTLEBELL

2C.

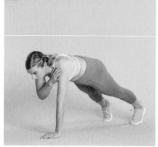
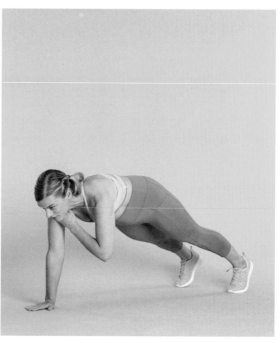

PLANK SHOULDER TAPS X 20

X3 SETS

3a.

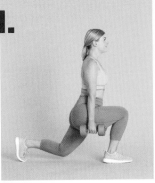

**SPLIT
LUNGES
X 8–10
EACH LEG**

2 X MEDIUM
DUMBBELLS

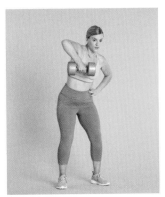

3b.

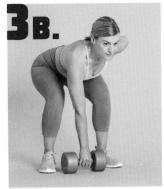

**SINGLE
ARM
DUMBBELL
SNATCHES
X 8–10
EACH ARM**

1 X MEDIUM
KETTLEBELL

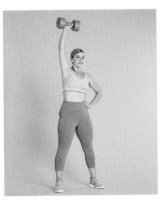

3c.

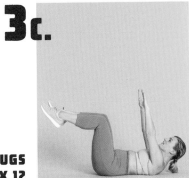

**DEADBUGS
X 12**

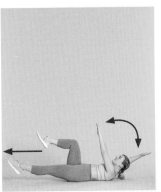

X3 SETS

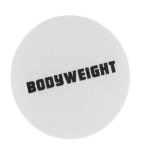

BODYWEIGHT

You'll need a chair (or bench/box if at the gym) for this one. We are doing a lower body circuit and an upper body circuit. **For each circuit, work for 40 seconds on, 20 seconds off and complete four rounds in total.** This week, we are shortening the rest period to 60 seconds between each round.

LOWER BODY CIRCUIT

SINGLE LEG STEP- UP (RIGHT)

SINGLE LEG STEP-UP (LEFT)

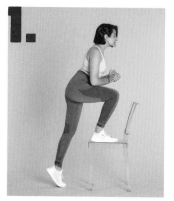

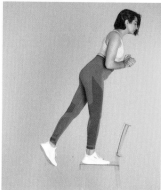

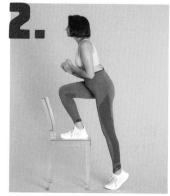

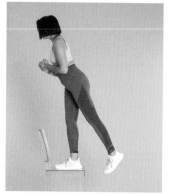

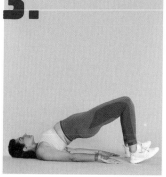

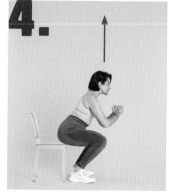

ELEVATED GLUTE BRIDGE

SEATED TO SQUAT JUMP

UPPER BODY CIRCUIT

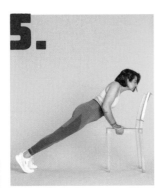

CHAIR PRESS-UPS

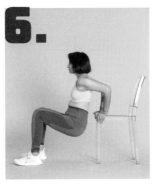

TRICEP DIPS

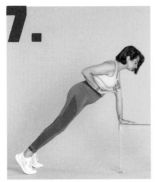

BODYWEIGHT PLANK ROWS

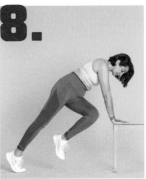

ELEVATED X-CLIMBER

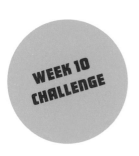

WEEK 10 CHALLENGE

Try for a new personal best! Have a go at re-testing your PB from week 5 and see how you get on, noting if it felt any easier or harder this time. Hopefully your workouts have been going well and if so your levels of overall strength and fitness should have increased. If you didn't get the result you expected in your chosen activity, consider how much your overall fitness, strength and stamina have improved over the past 10 weeks! I imagine you've been lifting heavier weights than you did on week 1?

Either way, I am super proud of you for putting your time and energy into building a strong foundation that I hope will support you in whatever you plan to do next on your fitness journey. It might be re-starting this 10-week programme and noticing how you have improved OR it may be on to something else. Either way, be PROUD of your efforts and celebrate every little victory on the way. You did it! Your body and mind are capable of great things.

REFERENCES

p.4 (1) Homan, K. J., & Tylka, T. L. 'Appearance-based exercise motivation moderates the relationship between exercise frequency and positive body image'. *Body Image* (2014) 11, 101–108

p.9 (2) www.mintel.com/press-centre/food-and-drink/brits-lose-count-of-their-calories-over-a-third-of-brits-dont-know-how-many-calories-they-consume-on-a-typical-day

p.10 (3) https://markets.businessinsider.com/news/stocks/245-billion-weight-loss-and-weight-management-market-2017-2022-by-equipment-surgical-equipment-diet-and-weight-loss-services-1005830884

pp.10–13 (4) Hall K.D., Kahan S. 'Maintenance of lost weight and long-term management of obesity'. *Medical Clinics of North America* (Jan 2018) 102(1):183–97

pp.10–13 (5) Anderson JW, Konz EC, Frederich RC, Wood CL. 'Long-term weight-loss maintenance: a meta-analysis of US studies'. *The American Journal of Clinical Nutrition*. (Nov 2001) 74(5):579–84

pp.10–13 (6) McEvedy SM, Sullivan-Mort G, McLean SA, Pascoe MC, Paxton SJ. 'Ineffectiveness of commercial weight-loss programs for achieving modest but meaningful weight loss: Systematic review and meta-analysis'. *Journal of Health Psychology*. (Oct 2017) 22(12):1614–27

pp.10–13 (7) Müller MJ, Enderle J, Bosy-Westphal A. 'Changes in energy expenditure with weight gain and Weight Loss in Humans'. *Current Obesity Reports*. (Dec 2016) 5(4):413–23

pp.10–13 (8) Müller M, Bosy-Westphal A, Heymsfield SB. 'Is there evidence for a set point that regulates human body weight?' *F1000 Medicine Reports*. (Aug 2010) 2:59

pp.10–13 (9) Stunkard AJ, Harris JR, Pedersen NL, McClearn GE. 'The Body-mass index of twins who have been reared apart'. *The New England Journal of Medicine* (May 1990) 322(21):1483–7

pp.10–13 (10) Dulloo AG, Jacquet J, Montani J-P, Schutz Y. 'How dieting makes the lean fatter: from a perspective of body composition autoregulation through adipostats and proteinstats awaiting discovery'. *Obesity Reviews* (Feb 2015) 16(S1):25–35

pp.10–13 (11) Sumithran P, Proietto J. 'The defence of body weight: a physiological basis for weight regain after weight loss'. *Clinical Science Journal* (Feb 2013) 124(4):231–41

pp.10–13 (12) Neumark-Sztainer D, Wall M, Larson NI, Eisenberg ME, Loth K. 'Dieting and disordered eating behaviors from adolescence to young adulthood: findings from a 10-year longitudinal study. *Journal of the American Dietetic Association*. (July 2011) 111(7):1004–11

pp.10–13 (13) Boyce JA, Kuijer RG. 'Focusing on media body ideal images triggers food intake among restrained eaters: A test of restraint theory and the elaboration likelihood model'. *Eating Behaviours Journal* (April 2014) 15(2):262–70

pp.10–13 (14) Goldschmidt AB, Wall M, Choo T-HJ, Becker C, Neumark-Sztainer D. 'Shared risk factors for mood-, eating-, and weight-related health outcomes'. *Journal of Health Psychology* (March 2016) 35(3):245–52

pp.10–13 (15) Dulloo AG, Montani J-P. 'Pathways from dieting to weight regain, to obesity and to the metabolic syndrome: an overview'. *Obesity Reviews* (Feb 2015) 16(S1):1–6

pp.10–13 (16) Mehta T, Smith DL, Muhammad J, Casazza K, Casazza K. 'Impact of weight cycling on risk of morbidity and mortality'. *Obesity Review* (Nov 2014) 15(11):870–81

pp.10–13 (17) Yeboah P, Hsu F-C, Bertoni AG, Yeboah J. 'Body mass index, change in weight, body weight variability and outcomes in type 2 diabetes mellitus' (from the ACCORD Trial). *The American Journal of Cardiology*. (2019 Feb) 123(4):576–81

pp.10–13 (18) Bhaskaran K, Dos-Santos-Silva I, Leon DA, Douglas IJ, Smeeth L. 'Association of BMI with overall and cause-specific mortality: a population-based cohort study of 3·6 million adults in the UK'. *Lancet Diabetes Endocrinol* (Dec 2018) 6(12):944–53.

pp.10–13 (19) Flegal KM, Kit BK, Orpana H, Graubard BI. 'Association of all-cause mortality with overweight and obesity using standard body mass index categories: a systematic review and meta-analysis'. JAMA. (Jan 2013) 309(1):71–82

pp.10–13 (20) Kramer CK, Zinman B, Retnakaran R. 'Are Metabolically Healthy Overweight and Obesity Benign Conditions?' *Annals of Internal Medicine* (Dec 2013);159(11):758

pp.10–13 (21) Matheson EM, King DE, Everett CJ. 'Healthy Lifestyle Habits and Mortality in Overweight and Obese Individuals'. J *American Board Family Medicine*. (Jan 2012) 25(1):9–15

pp.10–13 (22) Kuznetsova D. 'Healthy places: Councils leading on public health' (2012)

pp.10–13 (23) https://foodfoundation.org.uk/wp-content/uploads/2019/02/The-Broken-Plate.pdf

P.16 (1) Shisslak, C.M, Crago, M.,& Eses, L.S. 'The Spectrum of eating disturbances'. *International journal of Eating Disorders* (1995) 18 (3), 209–219

p.19 (2) Posner, J., Russell, J. A., & Peterson, B. S. 'The circumplex model of affect: an integrative approach to affective neuroscience, cognitive development, and psychopathology'. *Development and psychopathology* (2005) 17(3), 715–34

p.19 (3) Dr Suzuki, Wendy. 'The brain-changing benefits of exercise' https://www.youtube.com/watch?v=BHYOFxzoKZE&t=1s Building mental health resilience

p.19 (4) Schuch, F. B., Vancampfort, D., Firth, J., Rosenbaum, S., Ward, P. B., Silva, E. S. & Fleck, M. P. 'Physical activity and incident depression: a meta-analysis of prospective cohort studies'. *American Journal of Psychiatry* (2018) appi-ajp.

p.20 (5) 'Yoga for anxiety and depression' https://www.health.harvard.edu/mind-and-mood/yoga-for-anxiety-and-depression

p.21 (6) Dr Suzuki, Wendy. 'The brain-changing benefits of exercise' https://www.youtube.com/watch?v=BHYOFxzoKZE&t=1s

p.21 (7) Zhou, Z. Fu, J et al. 'Association between exercise and risk of dementia: results from a nationwide longitude study in China'. *BMJ open* (2017) 7 (12)

p.23 (8) Homan, K. J., & Tylka, T. L. 'Appearance-based exercise motivation moderates the relationship between exercise frequency and positive body image'. *Body Image* (2014) 11, 101–108

p.23 (9) Gilchrist, J. D., Pila, E., Castonguay, A., Sabiston, C. M., & Mack, D. E. 'Body pride and physical activity: Differential associations between fitness- and appearance-related pride in young adult Canadians'. *Body Image* (2018) 27, 77–85

p.30 (10) de Vries, D. A., Peter, J., de Graaf, H., & Nikken, P. 'Adolescents' social network site use, peer appearance-related feedback, and body dissatisfaction: testing a mediation model'. *Journal of Youth and Adolescence* (2016) 45(1), 211–224

p.30 (10) Holland, G., & Tiggemann, M. 'A systematic review of the impact of the use of social networking sites on body image and disordered eating outcomes'. *Body Image* (2016). 17, 100–110

p.31 (11) Cohen, R., Newton-John, T., & Slater, A. 'Selfie-objectification: The role of selfies in self-objectification and disordered eating in young women'. *Computers in Human Behavior* (2018) 79, 68–74

p.31 (11) Meier, E. P., & Gray, J. 'Facebook photo activity associated with body image disturbance in adolescent girls'. *Cyberpsychology, Behavior, and Social Networking* (2014) 17(4), 199–206

p.31 (12, 13) Cohen, R., Fardouly, J., Newton-John, T., & Slater, A. '#BoPo on Instagram: An experimental investigation of the effects of viewing body positive content on young women's mood and body image'. *New Media & Society* (2019)

p.31 (14) Slater, A., Varsani, N., & Diedrichs, P. C. '#fitspo or #loveyourself? The impact of fitspiration and self-compassion Instagram images on women's body image, self-compassion, and mood'. *Body Image* (2017) 22, 87–96

p.31 (15) Swami, V., Barron, D., Weis, L., & Furnham, A. Bodies in nature: 'Associations between exposure to nature, connectedness to nature, and body image in US adults'. *Body Image* (2016) 18, 153–161

p.32 (17) Tiggemann, M., & Zaccardo, M. 'Strong is the new skinny: A content analysis of #fitspiration images on Instagram'. *Journal of Health Psychology* (2018) 23(8), 1003–1011

p.32 (17) Tiggemann, M., & Zaccardo, M. 'Exercise to be fit, not skinny: The effect of fitspiration imagery on women's body image'. *Body Image* (2015) 15, 61–67

p.32 (18) Robinson, L., Prichard, I., Nikolaidis, A., Drummond, C., Drummond, M., & Tiggemann, M. (2017). 'Idealised media images: The effect of fitspiration imagery on body satisfaction and exercise behaviour'. *Body Image* (2019) 22, 65–71

p.32 (19) Hausenblas, H. A., & Fallon, E. A. 'Exercise and body image: A meta-analysis'. *Psychology and Health* (2006) 21(1), 33–47

p.32 (20) Homan, K. J., & Tylka, T. L. 'Appearance-based exercise motivation moderates the relationship between exercise frequency and positive body image'. *Body image* (2014). 11(2), 101–108
p.32 (21) Campbell, A., & Hausenblas, H. A. 'Effects of exercise interventions on body image: A meta-analysis'. *Journal of health psychology* (2009) 14(6), 780–793

p.32 (22) Homan, K. J., & Tylka, T. L. 'Appearance-based exercise motivation moderates the relationship between exercise frequency and positive body image'. *Body Image* (2014) 11(2), 101–108

p.32 (23) Tylka, T. L., & Homan, K. J. 'Exercise motives and positive body image in physically active college women and men: Exploring an expanded acceptance model of intuitive eating'. *Body Image* (2015) 15, 90–97

p.32 (24) Grogan, S. 'Body image and health: Contemporary perspectives'. *Journal of health psychology* (2006) 11(4), 523–530

p.32 (25¬¬) Fredrickson, B. L., & Roberts, T. A. 'Objectification theory: Toward understanding women's lived experiences and mental health risks'. *Psychology of Women Quarterly* (1997) 21(2), 173–206

p.32 (26) De Vries, D. A., & Peter, J. 'Women on display: The effect of portraying the self online on women's self-objectification'. *Computers in Human Behavior* (2013) 29(4), 1483–1489

p.33 (27, 28). Cohen, R., Fardouly, J., Newton-John, T., & Slater, A. '#BoPo on Instagram: an experimental investigation of the effects of viewing body positive content on young women's mood and body image'. *New Media & Society* (2019)

p.33 (29) Slater, A., Varsani, N., & Diedrichs, P. C. '#fitspo or# loveyourself? The impact of fitspiration and self-compassion Instagram images on women's body image, self-compassion, and mood'. *Body Image* (2017) 22, 87–96

p.35 (1) https://markets.businessinsider.com/news/stocks/245-billion-weight-loss-and-weight-management-market-2017-2022-by-equipment-surgical-equipment-diet-and-weight-loss-services-1005830884

p.38 (2) Tribole, Evelyn 'Intuitive Eating: research update'. SCAN (summer 2017)

p.43 (3) Smith T, Hawks S. 'Intuitive eating, diet composition, and the meaning of food in healthy weight promotion'. *Am J Health Educ.* (May/June 2006) 130–134

p.43 (4) Bruce L, Ricciardelli L. 'A systematic review of the psychosocial correlates of intuitive eating among adult women'. *Appetite* (2016) 96:454–472

p.43 (5) https://www.trusselltrust.org/news-and-blog/latest-stats/end-year-stats/

p.45 (1) Clifford, Dawn; Ozier, Amy; Bundros, Joanna; Moore, Jeffrey; Kreiser, Anna; Neyman Morris, Michelle 'Impact of non-diet approaches on attitudes, behaviors, and health outcomes: a systematic review' (2015)

p.49 (2) Engeln, Renee; Shavlik, Margaret; Daly, Colleen. 'Tone it down: how fitness instructors' motivational comments shape women's body satisfaction'. *Journal of Clinical Sport Psychology* (2018); Vol 12, issue 4, 508–524

p.51 (3) Chong Do, Lee; Blair, Steven N.; Jackson, Andrew S., 'Cardiorespiratory fitness, body composition, and all-cause and cardiovascular disease mortality in men' *American Journal of Clinical Nutrition* 69, no.3 (1999): 373–80

p.52 (4) Kumar et al. Journal of Back and Musculoskeletal Rehabilitation (2015) vol. 28, no. 4, 699–707

p.52 (5) Chang WD, Lin HY, Lai PT. 'Core strength training for patients with chronic low back pain'. J Phys Ther Sci. (2015) 27(3):619–622

p. 52 (6) Ohamad, Chan; Ebby Waqqash; Adnan Rahmat; Azmi, Ridzuan. 'Effectiveness of core stability training and dynamic stretching in rehabilitation of chronic low back pain patient'. *Malaysian Journal of Movement, Health & Exercise* (January 2019) [S.I.], v. 8, n. 1 ISSN 2600–9404

p.52 (7) Benedetti MG, Furlini G, Zati A, Letizia Mauro G. 'The Effectiveness of Physical Exercise on Bone Density in Osteoporotic Patients'. Biomed Res Int (2018)

p.60 (8) Williams, D. M., Dunsiger, S., Emerson, J. A., Gwaltney, C. J., Monti, P. M., & Miranda Jr, R. 'Self-paced exercise, affective response, and exercise adherence: a preliminary investigation using ecological momentary assessment'. *Journal of Sport and Exercise Psychology* (2016) 38(3), 282–291

p.60 (9) Rhodes, R. E., & Kates, A. 'Can the affective response to exercise predict future motives and physical activity behavior? A systematic review of published evidence'. *Annals of Behavioral Medicine* (2015) 49(5), 715–731

p.77 (10) Walker, Mathew *Why We Sleep* (2017) p. 107

p.77 (11) M.D Milewski et al 'Chronic lack of sleep is associated with increased sports injuries in adolescent athletes' Journal of Pediatric Orthopaedics (2014) 34, no.2 129–33

p.80 (12) De Barra, Micheal, Kimmo Eriksson, and Pontus Strimling. 'How Feedback biases give ineffective medical treatments a good reputation.' Journal of Medical Internet Research (2014): 16.9 e193.

RESOURCES

BOOKS

Body Respect by Linda Bacon and Lucy Aphramor
Health At Every Size by Linda Bacon

Just Eat It by Laura Thomas
Intuitive Eating by Evelyn Tribole and Elyse Resch
*The F*ck It Diet* by Caroline Dooner

Is Butter A Carb? by Rosie Saunt & Helen West

Beauty Sick by Renee Engeln
Beyond Beautiful by Anuschka Rees
Body Positive Power by Megan Jayne Crabbe
Happy Fat by Sofie Hagen

Big Fit Girl by Louise Green
Eat, Sweat, Play by Anna Kessel

Healthy Brain, Happy Life by Wendy Suzuki
Why We Sleep by Matthew Walker
The Gifts of Imperfection by Brené Brown
Daring Greatly by Brené Brown

PODCASTS

Nutrition Matters Podcast – Paige Smathers
Don't Salt My Game – Laura Thomas
The BodyLove Project – Jessi Haggerty
Food Psych Podcast – Christy Harrison
The Mindful Dietitian – Fiona Sutherland
Stronger Minds – Kimberley Wilson
The Strong Women Podcast – Hollie Grant
Fit & Fearless – Me, Zanna Van Dijk, Victoria Spence
Therapy Thoughts – Tiffany Roe
Unpacking Weight Science – Fiona Willer
The Food Medic Podcast – Dr Hazel Wallace

SOCIAL MEDIA ACCOUNTS

@tallyrye (me!)
@evelyntribole
@heytiffanyroe
@laurathomasphd
@therootedproject
@thephitcoach
@banhass
@aliceliveing
@lucymountain

@lucysheridan
@thedietboycott
@the.intuitive.trainer
@nudenutritionrd
@drjoshuawolrich
@scarrednotscared
@bodyposipanda
@calliethorpe

INDEX

ACKNOWLEDGEMENTS

I didn't think writing a book was on the cards for me, but when asked if I had something to say, I realized that I did. Ending the fight against my own body and freeing up the space in my brain it was consuming has enabled me to put that time and energy into writing this book, which I hope will help end the internal struggle for others too.

A big thank you to Helen West and Laura Thomas for planting the seed.

A big thank you to my grandma for providing the perfect writer's retreat.

Huge thanks to Jack, mum, Lydia, Isaac and my wonderful friends (you know who you are) for believing I could do this, giving great advice and letting me vent when I doubted myself.

Thank you to my team at Pavilion who took a risk on a different kind of fitness book and helped bring my vision to life. Thanks to Stephanie Milner, Laura Russell, Alice Sambrook and Katie Cowan for letting me be hands on and trusting my judgement.

CONTRIBUTORS
A massive thank you must also go to each person who helped make this book happen by sharing their expertise and insights. I utterly admire and respect each person, please go and check out their work:

Laura Thomas: laurathomasphd.co.uk
Dr. Sarah Vohra: themindmedic.co.uk
Kristina Bruce: kristinabruce.com
Anuschka Rees: anuschkarees.com
Nadia Craddock: podcasts.apple.com/gb/
podcast/appearance-matters-the-podcast/
id1069856498

Jessi Haggerty: jessihaggerty.com
Hollie Grant: pilatespt.co.uk/
Jonelle Lewis: movementformodernlife.
com/yoga-teacher/jonellelewis

MODELS
I am so grateful to each of the models for being part of the workout guide!
Please check out these incredible people:

Artika Gunathasan instagram.com/
artiliftsandeatsalot
Georgina Horne fullerfigurefullerbust.com
Devinia Noel devinianoel.com
Kaoutar Hannach evolvewithk.com

Gaby
Izzy
Sharan
Poppy

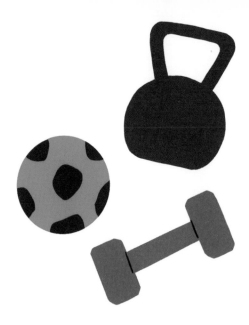

First published in the United Kingdom in 2020 by
Pavilion
43 Great Ormond Street
London
WC1N 3HZ

ISBN 978-1-911641-52-0

A CIP catalogue record for this book is available from the British Library.

10 9 8 7 6 5 4 3 2 1

Reproduction by Rival Colour Ltd, UK
Printed and bound by Toppan Leefung Printing Ltd, China

www.pavilionbooks.com

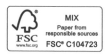